LEARNING
in the
COMMUNITY

LEARNING TO CARE
in the
COMMUNITY

Pat Turton
MSc, BSc, SRN, NDN CERT, RNT
Lecturer in Nursing, University of Manchester
and
Community Nursing Specialist (HIV/AIDS)
Regional Infectious Diseases Unit
Monsall Hospital, Manchester

Jean Orr
MSc, BA, RGN, HV Tutors Cert
Professor of Nursing Studies
The Queen's University of Belfast

With Co-authors
Joy Merrell
MSc, BSc (Hons), RGN, RHV, RNT, HV Tutors Cert
Lecturer in Nursing
University of Manchester
Brian Pateman
MA, DIP N (Lond), FETC, RGN, DN, PWT, DNT
Teaching Fellow
University of Manchester

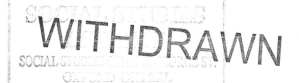
Edward Arnold
A member of the Hodder Headline Group
LONDON   MELBOURNE   AUCKLAND

© 1993 P Turton and J Orr

First published in Great Britain 1985
Second edition 1993

British Library Cataloguing in Publication Data

Turton, Pat
  Learning to Care in the Community. –
  2Rev.ed
  I. Title   II. Orr, Jean   III. Merrell, Joy
  IV. Pateman, Brian
  362.10425

  ISBN 0–340–55785–0

Typeset in 10/11 pt Times by Anneset, Weston-super-Mare, Avon.
Printed and bound in Great Britain for Edward Arnold, a division of Hodder
Headline PLC, Mill Road, Dunton Green, Sevenoaks, Kent TN13 2YA by
Biddles Ltd, Guildford and King's Lynn.

Contents

Editors' foreword

In most professions there is a traditional gulf between theory and its practice, and nursing is no exception. The gulf is perpetuated when theory is taught in a theoretical setting and practice is taught by the practitioner.

This inherent gulf has to be bridged by students of nursing, and the publication of this series is an attempt to aid such bridge building.

It aims to help relate theory and practice in a meaningful way whilst underlining the importance of the person being cared for.

It aims to introduce students of nursing to some of the more common problems found in each new area of experience in which they will be asked to work.

It aims to de-mystify some of the technical language they will hear, putting it in context, giving it meaning and enabling understanding.

Many thanks to Catherine Owens for the typing and preparation of the manuscript.

Acknowledgements

The publishers would like to thank the following for permission to use copyright material:

The British Medical Journal for Elliot, J. 1987: *ABC of AIDS: Nursing Care* and Barton, S.E. 1989: *Alternative Treatments for HIV Infection*. The Department of Health for Butters, E., Higginson *et al*. 1991: *Community HIV AIDS Teams* in Health Trends. HMSO Publications for Field, F. 1989: *House of Commons: AIDS Social Services Committee*. Journal of Palliative Care for Graydon, D. 1988: *AIDS: Observations of a Hospital Chaplain*. Open University Press for Smith, N. 1992: *Organising Support for Workers* in Reflective Helping in HIV and AIDS. Primary Health Care for Edwards, D. 1992: *A Team Spirit. A Model of Community Care for People with Late Stage HIV*. Professional Nurse for Irwin, R. 1992: *Homophobia in Health Care*. The Centre for Health Services Research, University of Newcastle upon Tyne for Bond, J., Rhodes, T. *et al*. 1988: *A National Study of HIV Infection, AIDS and Community Nursing Staff in England*.

Every effort has been made to trace copyright holders of material reproduced in this book. Any rights not acknowledged here will be acknowledged in subsequent printings if notice is given to the publisher.

Preface

Since this book was first published in 1985 there have been many changes in nursing and health care. The changes in nursing education known as Project 2000 have meant that nurse education now places emphasis on students being supernumary and students being no longer part of the workforce. The Project 2000 curriculum has had a major shift in emphasis to health and community. Diplomates from these courses are expected to be able to function as a first level nurse both in hospital and community and this is a development which is very exciting and welcomed. Many Project 2000 programmes start with students being in the community and having to understand not only the role of community nurses but also the economic, social and political effects of community on health and social care. Traditionally students would have spent three to four weeks in the community but now many are spending months in the community both in the Common Foundation Programme and in the Branch Programmes and of course for branches such as Mental Health and Mental Handicap much of the care is given in the community in any case. It is our view, however, that this book attempts to provide students with sufficient information to enable them to ask pertinent questions and to recognise what they are able to observe within the wider context of community. The emphasis in the book, as in the first edition, is largely on the Health Visitor and District Nurse, although there is an increased emphasis on the role of the practice nurse. In addition, we have included a chapter on nursing patients with HIV and AIDS in the community as this has been a major change since the book was first published.

This book is primarily written for students of nursing but it is also relevant to other people who are interested in understanding the provision of health care in the community. We do not look at the managerial or resource problems of those who are engaged in providing the services and we can only at this stage allude to the sorts of changes which might take place as a result of the National Health Service and Community Care reforms. There is no doubt however that students in the community will be seeing a much more fragmented and diverse service and that one of the major roles of nurse teachers will be to assist students in learning about the changing nature of health and social provision.

It appears that it will no longer be possible to make blanket statements about the provision of health care and community nursing care in particular as we move to the purchaser-provider split. What we have attempted to do however is to provide students with a baseline of what is going on in the community and to highlight the particular roles of community nurses as we move into the 1990s.

1 The Community

As a student undertaking community experience you may feel rather bewildered by the range of services which make up health and social care in the community. However, you have had experience of living in and being a member of various communities.

There are a wide range of services and different settings in which care is given in the community, depending on local needs. For example an inner city area will present different problems than a widespread rural farming community.

Background to changes in community care

Care in the community and health services provision to the community has been greatly affected by the National Health Service and Community Care Act of 1990. At the time of preparing this edition we have not had the opportunity to fully see the implications of these changes. The renewed emphasis on effectiveness, efficiency and quality control has led to the emergence of different models of health care, eg some hospitals and community units have opted for NHS Trust Status and general managers are now firming up contracts to provide services to a variety of purchasers. The result of the G.P. Contract has meant that there has been a rise in the number of Practice Nurses and the work of the General Practitioner is being increasingly focused on health promotion and prevention. Under the G.P. fundholding arrangements, fundholding practices will have to place contracts for community nursing services with providers of health care, although they will not be able to employ these staff directly and District Health Authorities will be the main link with social services. It may be when you are out in the community that the District Nurses and Health Visitors you meet will be working for G.P. fundholders although some may still be working with the Community Unit. In addition, there is a growing awareness of the importance of the public health function of health visitors and the G.P. fundholding contract will have to include some recognition of this important work.

It is important at this stage to say a little about what is meant by public health. Draper (1991) sets out the key issues for health through public policy and shows the link between health and economics and the wider community. He says that there are six general characteristics of the new public health:

1. Several sectors are often involved in a given health area and therefore health has a multi-sectorial focus.
2. Health policy needs to involve commerce and industry, voluntary organisations and the general public as well as central and local government.
3. Health hazards are not confined within national and regional boundaries.
4. The aim of health policy is to be educational and persuasive rather than dictatorial and puritanical.
5. Community health initiatives are an important part of health policy.
6. Health public policy is intrinsically political but not party political.

By this you can see that Draper is placing health in a much wider context than so far in hospital care. Allied to the emphasis on the new public health there have been a number of initiatives led by WHO, Healthy Cities is one which you might see in the community. Ashton and Seymour (1985) see the Healthy Cities project as a new European WHO initiative which is intended to lend support to city based health promotion. The project has its origins in the World Health Organisation's strategy of Health For All By The Year 2000 and is based on the 38 European Targets for Health For All. The European project is a collaborative one between the health promotion and environmental health sectors of WHO. It has particular emphasis on the promotion of healthy environments and lifestyles. The role of WHO in the project will be to act as a catalyst with facilitators in the process of agenda setting, consciousness raising and establishing models of good practice.

WHO says that Community Nurses acting as advocates for the community should help in the essential task of involving people in making decisions about health care and speaking for people's interests. Despite the many statements about health promotion it is still the case that most money and personnel go to the acute sector and this militates against the achievement of the Health For All goals. However, it is important as you are working in the community that you understand what the focus of the targets for Health For All are and these are as follows.

Focus of 'targets for health for all' by the year 2000 in Europe (WHO, 1986)

Targets 1–12: Health for all

1. Equity in health
2. Adding years to life
3. Better opportunities for the disabled
4. Reducing disease and disability
5. Eliminating measles, polio, neonatal tetanus, congenital rubella, diphtheria, congenital syphilis and indigenous malaria
6. Increased life expectation at birth
7. Reduced infant mortality
8. Reduced maternal mortality
9. Combating disease of the circulation
10. Combating cancer
11. Reducing accidents
12. Stopping the increase in suicide

Targets 13–17: Lifestyles conducive to health for all

13. Developing healthy public policies
14. Developing social support systems
15. Improving knowledge and motivation for healthy behaviour
16. Promoting positive health behaviour
17. Decreasing health-damaging behaviour

Targets 18–25: Producing healthy environments

18. Policies for healthy environments
19. Monitoring, assessment and control of environmental risks
20. Controlling water pollution
21. Protecting against air pollution
22. Improving food safety
23. Protecting against hazardous wastes
24. Improving housing conditions
25. Protecting against work-related health risks

Targets 26–31: Providing appropriate care

26. A health care system based on primary health care
27. Distribution of resources according to need
28. Re-orientating primary medical care
29. Developing teamwork
30. Co-ordinating services
31. Ensuring quality of services

Targets 32–38: Support for health development

32. Developing a research base for health for all
33. Implementing policies for health for all
34. Management and delivery of resources
35. Health information systems
36. Training and deployment of staff
37. Education of people in non-health sectors
38. Assessment of health technologies

The Health of the Nation (DOH, 1991) document is a discussion paper produced by the Government which demonstrates an interest in and focus on prevention and targeting, and sets the agenda for preventive health care in the future. Some of the health areas identified include the prevention of coronary heart disease and stroke, cancer, smoking, eating and drinking, prevention of accidents, health of pregnant women and children, diabetes, mental health, rehabilitation and asthma. The Government has gone on to identify some key areas and has issued a subsequent document called **The Health of the Nation – First Steps for the NHS** (NHS Management Executive, 1992) and this document highlights the areas that should have particular priority and the levels of service which have an important role to play. The issues they have identified for which targets will be set are coronary heart disease and stroke, cancers, mental illness, HIV/AIDS and sexual health, and accidents. To give you an example of the type of approach that is being taken we will look at what primary health care is being asked to do in terms of coronary heart disease and stroke:

Suggestions for primary health care

- Development of protocols for detection, diagnosis and management of patients with hypertension (in discussion with secondary care).
- Consider providing education and advice on diet, smoking, salt intake, exercise and alcohol.
- Consider need for access to dietetic expertise, aiming to ensure adequate nutrition education and training for all appropriate professionals and other staff.
- Development of policy for preventing the recurrence of stroke/TIA, and myocardial infarction.
- Development of policies for the management of stroke/TIA, chest pain and CHD, including referral guidelines agreed between primary and secondary care.
- Consider developing practice profiles to include information on smoking and alcohol intake.
- It is recommended that ante-natal clinics offer smoking cessation advice and support to pregnant women.

- Consider adopting healthy workplace initiatives including policy on smoking, healthy eating and alcohol, and counselling, advice and awareness raising (including access to exercise).

These are the types of initiatives that community nurses will be able to contribute to and many of these changes have of course highlighted the important role that nursing has to play not just in looking after people who are ill but in preventive work and in the important area of rehabilitation.

Health care does not of course stand alone and within the NHS and Community Care Act there are radical changes proposed for the provision of social care in the community. This will be in operation by 1993 and will mean that nurses will be involved in the assessment and care management of clients in the community and that packages of care will be drawn up in an attempt to maintain people in their own homes. This will involve much more inter-sectoral cooperation, multi-disciplinary work with colleagues in social service departments as well as general practitioners and voluntary agencies. When you are out in the community you need to be aware of the changes taking place in the work of Health Visitors and District Nurses to accommodate this important change in the provision for those in need.

In whatever setting you are working it is necessary to consider:

1 What is meant by Community?
2 What is Community Care?
3 How do we assess Community Health Needs?
4 Key influences on health.

What is meant by community?

The word community poses problems of definition. Let's think of the many ways the word is used. We talk of community nursing, community policing, community spirit, community groups and community education. In nursing we utilise the word in two main ways. Firstly we use it to describe the location of activities e.g. community nursing. Secondly we use it to place value or worth on feelings and sentiments, e.g. we speak of community spirit to describe the feelings shared by people within a particular region.

It is likely that you think of the community in which you live in terms of two elements. Firstly you identify the community as a place and secondly, as a set of relationships which are important to you, e.g. neighbours. In the first we are referring to a defined geographical area; we need to study those aspects of the environment which are its features. In the second we are referring to the social relationships and networks which exist within the area and which contribute to the lives of the residents. Can you outline the important geographical and environmental characteristics of your community? For example which of the characteristics mentioned in Fig 1.1 most influence how you feel about your community?

Which of the social relationships and networks do you think are important in your life and the local groups and organisations you use: family, relatives, friends, local organisations?

When we talk of assessing the community therefore, we are focussing on these two elements, both of which are important for the health of the residents and the type of community care which is available.

What is community care?

In the 1950 to 1960's there was a move to encourage hospitals and local health authorities to adopt policies which would maintain people in the community instead of in large institutions. In part this was because community care was thought to be cheaper and in addition there was a growing concern at the standards of care given in large institutions. It was also felt that people preferred to be out of hospital. Although the philosophy of care in the community was adopted, there is no agreed definition of what is meant by it.

Community care can mean care provided in peoples' own home by a range of health and social services such as District Nurses and home helps. In addition voluntary bodies such as Age Concern provide some services to supplement those provided by the state.

Community care can also mean care by health and social service

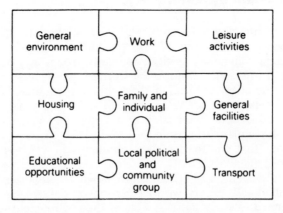

Fig. 1.1 Environmental features of a community

workers in residential accommodation, which is small scale and situated within the local community. Examples of this are hostels for the mentally handicapped and old peoples' homes. Sheltered accommodation for elderly people may be provided by Social Services and the Housing Department.

Examples of health and social services for the elderly: District Nurses, home helps, Health Visitors, chiropodists, General Practitioners, occupational therapists, meals on wheels, day centres, social workers and voluntary organisations (e.g. Help the Aged).

These two types of community care can be described as '*Care in the Community*'. There is a third type which is best described as '*Care by the Community*'. This means care given by family, relatives, friends and neighbours. In other words, care given by the support systems which exist within an area. Despite the help offered by the health and social services it is this type of care, outlined in Fig. 1.2, which is often fundamental to maintaining people in the community.

These systems often exist together. For example, a mentally handicapped child may be cared for largely by the family and relatives with help from Health Visitors, social workers and voluntary bodies such as the National Society for Mentally Handicapped Children.

Care given by the community often means care given by women, i.e. neighbours, mothers and daughters, and the services assume these carers have a responsibility to care for the elderly and chronic disabled within the family and the community. The stresses of this type of caring are seldom recognised. Many women have to combine

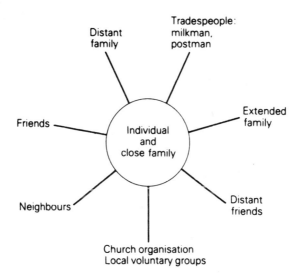

Fig. 1.2 Social support system in the community

work outside the home with the responsibility of caring for dependants and therefore, any reductions in the health and social services affect these women most acutely and impose great strain on family life. In addition it may be that the carers, friends and relatives are themselves elderly and frail and can find the effort required damaging to their own health.

So far we have described community care which exists for those with health or social problems. There are, however, a range of preventive services to help people remain healthy, and to which people can go for the treatment of minor ailments or to be referred to hospital services.

Examples of preventive health services: Health Visitors, community midwives, Community Psychiatric Nurses, Family Planning, cytology clinics, well women clinics, immunisation programmes, child health clinics, school health services, General Practitioners, dental services, speech therapists, physiotherapy, occupational therapy, Health Education Departments and chemists.

It must be stressed that many people seek counsel from friends and relatives on health matters and use the chemist as a source of advice and treatment. As shown by Fig. 1.3, it has been said that only the tip of the iceberg of illness is seen by G.P.'s. The submerged part is made up of people treating themselves or getting help from occupational health services or the range of voluntary organisations which are a feature of the British health and welfare system. Public libraries have information on local and national voluntary bodies. Also try the phone book, library, Citizens Advice Bureau, local clinic or social services offices.

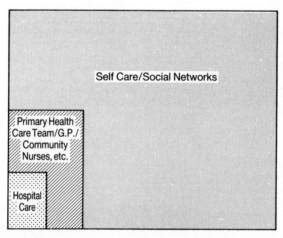

Fig. 1.3   Amount of care given by different sources

Examples of sources of help in the community: Age Concern, Alcoholics Anonymous, British Diabetic Association, Gingerbread (for one parent families), local church groups, Good Neighbour Schemes, marriage guidance, Mind (National Association for Mental Health), Multiple Sclerosis Society, Pregnancy Advisory Service, Royal National Institute for the Blind, Royal National Institute for the Deaf and the Samaritans.

Where to go for help in the community

Your local social services for a social worker, Day Centres, Day Nurseries, Luncheon Clubs, a place in a home, Meals on Wheels, a home help, aids for the disabled, Travel Permits for the disabled, a Welfare Rights Officer.

Housing Aid Centre for advice on rent, help for homeless, help with housing and landlord/tenant problems.

Citizens Advice Bureaux for information and advice on Legal Aid schemes, unemployment problems, Hire Purchase problems, consumer problems, tribunal appeals, personal problems, financial problems.

Community Health Council which is an independent body providing information and advice on hospital and clinic services, family practitioner services, i.e. G.P.'s, Dentists, Chemists, Opticians, etc., complaints procedures.

Local Education Authority offices for free school meals, maintenance grants, school clothing grants, bus fare refunds and bus passes.

Social Security Benefits Offices for national insurance benefits, supplementary pensions and allowances, family income supplements, help with prescriptions, dental treatment and glasses, free milk and vitamins and benefits for the disabled.

Welfare Rights Officers for advice and help with all benefit problems.

Law Centres for legal advice for tenants and council tenants, on welfare rights except supplementary benefits, on employment problems and minority group rights.

Council for Voluntary Service (CVS) for help with a wide range of voluntary services.

Local Authority Housing Department for rent and rate rebates and rent allowances.

Community Health Services for antenatal, chiropody, home nursing, Health Visitors, family planning and well women clinics, school dental, nursing and family guidance services.

Assessing community health needs

Assessing the health needs of a community involves a number of approaches. Firstly we need to get the feel of the area and then examine certain aspects in depth. Much of this information can be obtained from the primary health care nurses working in the community but first of all see what *you* think of the community in which you are working.

Getting to know the area

This is your first time in a new community. Spend some time getting the feel of what it must be like to reside in this area and what factors are important for health and health care. Throughout the day spend time visiting shops, walking around the streets, visiting cafes, leisure centres and libraries. See who is queueing at the Post Office; is it mainly young mothers or elderly people? Are there young people hanging around street corners? What type of people are in the streets? Are they friendly? Would you like to live here? It is very important that you ask local people how they feel about their community and what they see as the major problems and advantages.

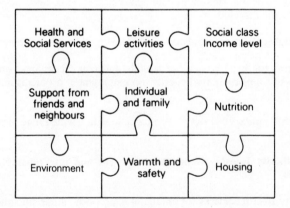

Fig. 1.4   Factors influencing health

Factors which influence health

After the initial assessment spend time examining the community in more depth.

- **Environment**
  What type of area is it? (e.g. inner city, rural, small village)
  Is it well kept or is there evident vandalism and graffitti?
  What facilities exist? (e.g. leisure centres and parks)
  What range of shops are present? (including chemist and Post Office)
  What is the transport system?
  Is the community isolated from main centres of shopping?
  What services exist for children?
  Are there any obvious health hazards? (e.g. canals or motorways and pollution from factories)
- **Housing**
  What types of housing are there?
  What is the condition of the housing?
  Are the houses near the shops and facilities?
  Is there play space for children?
  Is there a local centre such as a community hall?
  Where is the library?
- **Health care facilities**
  Where is the local clinic in relation to housing?
  Is there a health centre?
  What services exist?
  Who uses the facilities?
  Where are the nearest hospitals especially Accident and Emergency Departments and antenatal clinics?
- **Social services and benefits office**
  Where is the local Social Services office?
  Where is the local benefits office?
  Is there sheltered housing/hostels?
  Is there a local job centre? What age of people use it?
  Are there day centres for elderly/mentally handicapped people?
- **Employment opportunities**
  What are the major industries nearby?
  Is there a high level of unemployment?
  Do people travel outside the area to work?
  What type of jobs are advertised in shops and newspapers?
- **Population structure**
  What is the breakdown of the area by age and sex?
  What groups are there who have special health needs? (e.g. minority ethnic groups).

- **Health status**
  What are major causes of death?
  What are the major types of illness?
  How many families are on 'at risk' registers for child abuse?
  What are the child-rearing patterns and how do they affect health?
  What families are in poor housing?

Having undertaken an assessment of the community health needs, we list the main areas of concern and plan action. As an example let us examine what activities might be undertaken if we found a high level of road traffic accidents, affecting children and elderly people, at a major road junction.

Expected outcomes – plan

To educate the community about the dangers of road traffic accidents.
To motivate residents to campaign for a safe crossing at the junction.

Action

- **Children**
  Contact local schools to organise a health education programme on accident prevention.
  Encourage the teachers to undertake project work on accidents.
  Undertake a health education programme in the local health centre, library and community halls.
  Encourage parents to be aware of accident prevention in the course of home visiting, and to write to local community representatives, radio and newspapers.
  Talk to children at local youth organisations.
- **Elderly people**
  Visit local day centres and talk about the problem.
  Raise the topic in home visiting to the elderly.
  Undertake a health education programme in the local health centre, Post Office and library.
  Encourage the elderly to write to local councillors, newspapers and radio.
- **General**
  Contact the Royal Society for Prevention of Accidents (ROSPA).
  Write to the local newspaper about the problem.
  Contact the local radio and newspaper with articles on road safety.
  Set up a health education stall in the main shopping area.

Evaluation

The level of accidents should be monitored for six months and the campaign reassessed in the light of the results.

Key influences on health

As we have seen there are many factors which influence health. We shall examine three in depth which have particular importance for primary health care nurses in the community. These are: housing and environment, the family and poverty.

Housing and environment

Provision of a healthy environment is of special concern to primary health care nurses. If a family lives in a deprived inner city area for example, it is likely that they will suffer from a number of deprivations which are interrelated (multiple deprivation). These include poor housing, few job opportunities, limited educational and recreational facilities and inadequate health care facilities. The crime and vandalism rate will be high and people may be afraid to go out at night and thus become isolated. The general environment of such areas tends to be unpleasant, with broken bottles, abandoned cars and few open spaces or parks and so there will be a high accident rate. We often view our home and surrounding area as an extension of ourselves and other people may judge us by where we live.

There is a strong relationship between housing and health. Poor housing conditions can affect families and influence the standards of child care. Overcrowding can limit the availability of privacy and cause stress and friction between family members.

Effects of housing on health:

The following diseases are related to poor housing:

- Acute respiratory infections due to inadequate heating and crowded sleeping conditions
- Parasite and intestinal infections due to inadequate washing and toilet facilities
- Home accidents due to bad lighting, dangerous wiring, crowded accommodation
- Infectious and non-infectious diseases of the skin related to inadequate washing facilities
- Infectious diseases of childhood
- Mental health due to overcrowding and stress

Focus on the family

The primary health care workers are concerned not only with the individual but with the family and the influence of the wider community on the family e.g. unemployment in the wider community may affect the job prospects of family members which in turn increases stress and leads to ill health. Family members are often the main providers of health care. Women play a major role in caring for ill relatives and neighbours and for maintaining family health in the areas of nutrition and hygiene. We need to assess the family because:

1 Any illness or problem affecting one family member will affect other members and can lead to problems for the family unit as a whole. For example, if a father is unemployed the family will be affected financially and also have to cope with him being at home all day.
2 The family unit is the main support for members who are under stress or are ill.
3 It is within our family that we learn behaviours which may lead to ill health.
4 Family members influence whether or not health services are used.
5 Family members share genetic traits e.g. cystic fibrosis
6 There is a relationship between early family experience and how healthy we are in terms of life styles we later adopt such as eating patterns.
7 Individuals' view of themselves is based on experiences within the family e.g. a child may have behaviour problems because of lack of attention from the parents.

The Health Visitor and District Nurse are involved with the family in a very close way, but what is meant by the term family and what types of families are you likely to see in the community? It is usual to talk of two main types of families – the nuclear family and the extended family.
Nuclear family. This is the family of marriage or parenthood, comprised of a woman and man and their children.
Extended family. This is the kinship networks of sisters, brothers, aunts, uncles, grandparents and cousins related to a family by marriage or parenthood.

There are many changes taking place in family life in Britain and it is difficult to talk about the 'typical family' which we often see on television advertising, of the mother at home, the working father and two children.

Family trends:

- Increase in one person households, typicaly elderly people and young people prior to marriage
- Increase in one parent families with dependant children
- Increase in cohabitation
- Increase in divorce (one out of every three marriages)
- Increase in remarriage

Despite these changes the family unit remains important for its members and society as a whole. The Health Visitor and District Nurse have to be aware of the different needs of the families in the caseload and how these families relate to the community. They have to take account of all the members of the family and outside influences on the family.

Poverty

There is a relationship between poverty and ill health and this has been documented in the Black Report on inequalities in health (Townsend, 1982). This report states for example that babies of unskilled manual parents are twice as likely to die within the first month of life compared to babies of parents who are in the professional classes. The poor are more likely to have diseases of the respiratory system, infective and parasitic diseases, to suffer from poor nutrition and to have 'small for date' babies. Poor children may suffer from nutritional diseases and are more at risk from accidents both in the home and in the surrounding area.

Groups in poverty: Low wage earners, elderly, chronically ill/handicapped, long-term unemployed, one parent families and those on long-term social security.

Changes in our social structure mean that there are now an increasing number of one parent families, many of whom live in poverty.

Test yourself

1 What voluntary organisations exist for elderly people in your community?
2 List the health services which exist in the health centre or clinic from which you work.
3 What self-help groups are available in the community?
4 What health education takes place in local schools?
5 What hospital/community liaison schemes exist in the community?

6   What occupational health services are offered by one local employer?
7   What are the main health needs of the community?
8   What changes are taking place in community nursing with the NHS Act?

2 The Primary Health Care Team

Like an amoeba our society and its health needs are constantly responding to epidemiological, demographic, ecological, political, economic and technological forces with the resulting changes in public attitudes and knowledge, as summarised in Fig. 2.1. *Consequently we live in a period when despite 'medical inflation', solutions are few and preventive care has become as important as cure.* This concern is reflected in government policies, which support a shift in emphasis and resources from hospital to community care; the burden of the resulting workload becomes the responsibility of the members of the Primary Health Care Team.

The concept of the Primary Health Care Team has been promoted extensively in the UK since the mid 1970s and although the concept's popularity has increased and decreased at different times it is still relevant today in the 1990s. Although the modern terms have changed and the talk may be of packages of care, shared visions, or seamless

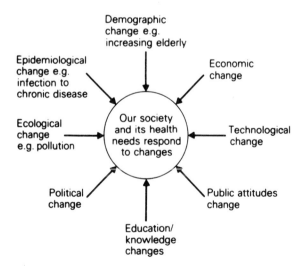

Fig. 2.1 Importance of care in a changing society

care, the basic philosophy of co-ordinated and co-operative working is as relevant today as ever.

Definitions:

A *team* is: 'a group of people who make different contributions towards the achievement of a common goal.'
A *Primary Health Care Team* is: 'an independent group of general medical practitioners, secretaries and/or receptionists, Health Visitors, District Nurses and midwives who share a common purpose and responsibility, each member clearly understanding his/her own function and those of the other members so that they all pool skills and knowledge to provide an effective primary health care service.'

Gilmore, Bruce & Hunt, 1974

The aims of primary health care are:

1   The promotion of health in its broadest terms, through education, support and the encouragement of self-care.
2   The prevention of ill health by prophylaxis, early diagnosis education and advice on the value of early contact with the primary health care services.
3   The care, treatment and rehabilitation of those who are acutely or chronically ill.
4   The referral of patients to specialist services where necessary, and the provision of continuing care following specialist treatment.

The means to achieve these aims is through the effective work of Primary Health Care Teams. (Source: Chief Nursing Officer, DHSS, 1977)

Teamwork in primary care is seen as the best way of meeting the challenge posed by the changes in the community's health needs.
Examples of these changes are:

1   The increasing numbers of elderly, many of whom may be ill and remain at home (demographic change).
2   Changes in family structure and greater geographical mobility which means fewer people available to care for their sick relatives and more single parent families.
3   Increasing problem of lifestyle diseases, e.g. heart disease, lung cancer, obesity (epidemiological change).
4   Changes in treatment policy, e.g. early discharge from hospital for surgical patients (political/technological change).
5   Limited resources available for the health care services, e.g. insufficient staff (political/economic change).

What makes the Primary Health Care Team different from other teams?

We have all had experiences of being a member of a team. It may have been in a hockey or netball team where the aim was to get as many goals as possible and each team member had a particular position and role to play but everyone is on the field together. Or it may have been in a swimming team where each member swims their race alone according to their particular skills e.g. backstroke or breaststroke and their points contribute towards their team's final score. The first example requires more membership co-operation than the second but both teams have a common goal i.e. to win, and decisions regarding strategy are taken together.

Within the community there is no agreed hierarchy, each of the main professions represented has a long history of working independently of each other, organising their own work, making their own decisions and taking responsibility for their actions. Thus teamwork in the community is providing co-ordinated action by a group of individual professions to achieve better care for patients.

Although the lack of a hierarchical structure has led to some problems e.g. duplication of actions, it is agreed by everyone that the standard of care given by a team is far better than that provided by any individual professional working alone!

Advantages of teamwork in primary care:

- Care given by a group is greater than the sum of individuals' care.
- Rare skills are used more appropriately.
- Peer influence and informal learning within the group raises the standards of care.
- Team members have increased job satisfaction.
- Team working encourages co-ordinated health education.
- Team working lowers the prevalence of disease in the community.
- The individual gets more efficient and understanding treatment when ill.

A patient being cared for at home may need the support and services of many different people from the team. These may include one or several of the following workers – Nurses, Midwives, Health Visitors, General Practitioners, Social Workers, Home Helps, Care Assistants, Physiotherapists, specialist nurses (e.g. stoma nurse), volunteers (e.g. meals on wheels staff).

The patient and carers may also be included as members of the Primary Health Care Team in that they are actively involved in deciding on the carrying out of care and treatment procedures.

Members of the team may be based together in a health centre or may work from different premises. Although ideally they are housed together this is not essential for good teamwork.

Functions of primary health care teams: Ambulant and domiciliary care, emergency care, screening, health education, medico-social care, identification of needs and identification of preventive measures required to maintain and improve the health of the community, teaching and research.

Who is a member of the Primary Health Care Team?

Which individuals or professionals are included in the team will depend on the particular task the team is organised to perform; the team may dissolve when the task is completed. This is exemplified by the tasks given in Fig. 2.2.

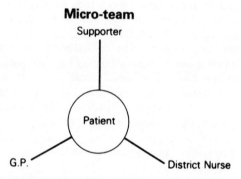

Fig. 2.2a Task: Management of a patient's acute illness at home: a follow-up visit to remove sutures

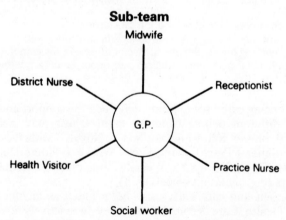

Fig. 2.2b Task: Management of family or community care

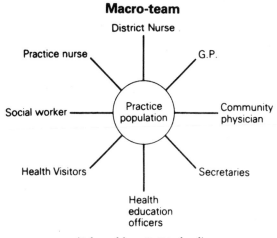

Macro-team

(Adapted from P. Pritchard)

Fig. 2.2c Task: Screening a practice population for a preventive health programme

The major health problems facing our society are what have been called the lifestyle diseases, e.g. heart disease, cancer (especially cancer of the lung), and stress-related conditions e.g. mental illness. In the past the health service tended to emphasise cure as opposed to prevention but it is now recognised that especially where the lifestyle diseases are concerned we should be concentrating on prevention. One of the most important functions, therefore of the Primary Health Care Team is in promoting health and preventing ill health.

Promoting health via health education

WHO (1969) set out what health education hopes to achieve: it aims (1) to persuade people to adopt and sustain healthful life practices, (2) to use the health service wisely and (3) to make their own decisions both individually and collectively to improve their health status and environment.

Health education means different things to different people – traditionally it has meant giving information about factors that promote physical health (e.g. stop smoking, diet) but it is now used in a much wider sense. Health education can be formal or informal and opportunities for the nurse to practice it are limitless. It must also must be remembered that nurses and doctors actions are noted by patients and these may have a great influence on their health behaviour. Much of this influence may be unintended and contrary to the desired health message, e.g. when a nurse is seen smoking other people may take this as evidence that smoking is really not that harmful.

Preventing ill health

The Primary Health Care Team is also concerned with preventing ill health but what is meant by the word prevention? There are three levels of prevention: primary, secondary and tertiary.

Primary prevention: before the disease process or disability has started. A potential problem or illness is anticipated and action is taken to avoid the condition. An example is the range of immunisation programmes which protect a population from diseases such as polio, measles and rubella. Another example would be giving advice to parents, children and elderly people on how to make their homes safe and thus cut down the risk of a home accident.

Secondary prevention: when illness/disability may still be alleviated or arrested. This includes early detection (e.g. screening), diagnosis and treatment of health problems. An example is motivating a client with dental caries to apply for dental treatment.

Tertiary prevention: when illness or disability has occurred and maintenance and rehabilitation is the aim. The damage resulting from a previous mental or physical illness or any chronic condition must be alleviated as much as possible. An example is helping a woman to deal with her feelings following a mastectomy to prevent depression. Often in tertiary prevention the emphasis is on rehabilitation.

Whilst you are out observing the work of different community nurses try to identify and classify preventive measures. What types of prevention have you heard being discussed when you visit with the Health Visitor and District Nurse?

The amount of time or the emphasis given to health education and prevention varies, however, depending on the role of the worker e.g. Health Visitor, District Nurse or G.P. The Health Visitor for example places the major importance on primary prevention and spends proportionately less time on secondary and tertiary prevention. The District Nurse on the other hand tends to emphasise secondary and tertiary prevention.

During your community experience you may visit and learn about a very wide range of health and social services provided in your particular area. Community experience is organised very differently from one school of nursing to another, but it is usual for all nurses to spend some time at least with the Health Visitors and the District Nurses. In this book, therefore, we have decided to concentrate on these two key members of the Primary Health Care Team and to consider the other services within the context of their work.

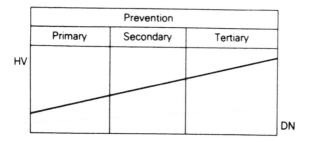

Fig. 2.3 Proportion of time spent on different aspects of prevention by a District Nurse (DN) and a Health Visitor (HV)

Nurses in the community

At the time of writing there is considerable organisational and philosophical changes taking place in community nursing. These changes are creating new opportunities and challenges for community nurses. This means that it is more difficult than in the previous edition of this book to clearly state the role and function of specific community nurses, as quite rightly their role is influenced by local need more than national or professional guidelines. The following descriptions are just an outline of the role of different nurses in the community, you may well find that your community nurse has a specialised role rather than a generalist one. In any case, to get the fullest picture of community nursing it is essential that you·compare and contrast your community nursing experience with your peers.

The major changes taking place are in the education, employment, and professional function of community nurses.

Education

Following the development of Project 2000 there was a need to examine post registration education and practice and the United Kingdom Council set up a sub-group to look at community nursing (UKCC, 1990). The outcome of this work is as follows:

Firstly, there is to be a new discipline of nurses to work in the community under the title of Community Health Care Nurses. This is seen as an overall title to describe the setting in which care takes place in much the same way as nurses on wards are called Hospital Nurses. It is envisaged that nurses in the community will keep the names that they already have as the titles of Health Visitor, District Nurse, etc. are familiar to the public.

Secondly, there will continue to be a range of nurses to meet the health care needs of society. The UKCC's report underlined the complexity of work that was undertaken in the community and recognised the need for well qualified nurses and health visitors with specialist skills in education.

Thirdly, the Project 2000 diplomat will be able to work as a first level nurse under the direction of a qualified Community Health Care Nurse. This reaffirms the view that there will need to be a system of further education in order to qualify nurses to work in the different specialties within the community.

Fourthly, the future preparation of Community Health Care Nurses will be based on the following criteria:

Credit for appropriate experience in education will be given. The courses will be modular and there will be shared learning. The design of the courses are to be flexible within the parameters determined by the UKCC and the programmes will be designed to meet the core skills of all Community Health Care Nurses with additional add-on modules for specific areas of practice.

The advantages of the proposals of the UKCC are seen to match clinical responsibility with tailored preparation in order to improve standards of care. The recording of the qualification in Community Health Care Nursing on the Register will protect standards and indicate skills.

The scheme should create a rational and cost effective framework to make more rational use of resources and provide a more flexible education relevant and responsible to health care services.

The future preparation for Community Health Care Nurses will focus on three main areas: clinical management and care management, programme management and team leadership.

Employment

Community nurses with the exception of practice nurses, who are employed by G.P.s, have been employees of the Health Authority. Potential employers and purchasers of community nurses services are now G.P.s, Health Authorities, Hospital or Independent Community Trusts, Family Health Service Authorities, and Local Authority Social Service Departments. Great variance in role is therefore possible.

Professional function of community nurses

There are two developments in community nursing which will change practice. The first is the trend towards greater autonomy accountability and removal of restrictions to practice which has been firmly outlined in the UKCC document 'The Scope of Professional Practice' (1992). The second development, Nurse Prescribing, follows this trend towards greater efficiency and professional accountability.

Nurse prescribing

Nurse prescribing was first officially suggested in Neighbourhood Nursing – A Focus For Care (DHSS, 1986). This wide ranging influential report is known to community nurses as the Cumberlege report after Julia Cumberlege who chaired the report. Recommendation 7 stated:

> The DHSS should agree a limited list of items and simple agents which may be prescribed by nurses as part of a nursing care programme, and issue guidelines to enable nurses to control drug dosage in well-defined circumstances.

The DHSS agreed with this statement and commissioned a working party chaired by Dr J Crown. The ensuing, Report Of The Advisory Group On Nurse Prescribing (DOH, 1989) stated that suitably qualified nurses working in the community, District Nurses and Health Visitors should be able to **prescribe** from a Nurses' Formulary. (The Nurses' Formulary is a list of items which a nurse can prescribe from the drug tariff and is the limited list mentioned in the Cumberlege report.) In addition, other nurses working in the community should be able to **supply** drugs, dressings and appliances under a locally agreed group protocol. Good examples of nurses who could supply would be stoma or continence advisers. The final area where the Crown Report recommended that nurses should be involved in prescribing was **adjusting** the timing and dosage of medicines within a patient specific protocol. Examples of nurses who are likely to be involved in adjusting dosage for a particular patient, in agreement with the medical practitioner who originally prescribed the treatment, would be diabetes nurses and those caring for the terminally ill.

Nurse prescribing is an example of multiskilling which means a professional takes on a small part of what has been traditionally exclusively another role enabling them to fulfil the needs of their patients more effectively. The other professional also benefits as there is greater opportunity to concentrate on those problems which require their knowledge and skills.

Nurse prescribing benefits both patients and the nurse. An example will demonstrate this. The G.P. would ask the district nurse to visit a patient and assess the wound and suggest appropriate treatment. Having seen the wound the nurse would request a prescription from the G.P., if the patient or relatives took this request to the G.P. they would inevitably have to wait until the next day for the actual prescription which they would then still have to take to the chemist. Not only is the whole procedure time consuming it is also professionally demeaning for both the nurse and the G.P. The nurse's expertise in wound care means that she is seen as fit to decide treatment but not to write the prescription. The G.P. by rubberstamping the nurse's prescription is accepting accountability for treatment given by another professional even though the other professional is managing this element of care.

As well as saving time, the ability to initially prescribe and alter timing and dosage of drugs is complimentary to good nursing practice. The care of the terminally ill provides a good example of how speedy and effective symptom control is an essential part of nursing care.

The ability of Health Visitors to prescribe means that minor problems noted at the child clinic can be dealt with there and then. For example a mother seeking advice about what she considers is simple nappy rash caused by an obvious fungal infection can be treated without the mother making another appointment to see the G.P.

An education programme set up to allow existing District Nurses and Health Visitors to become nurse prescribers is intended to be completed by 1995. Nurse prescribing has been postponed at present but it is hoped that it will come on stream in the near future. However, there is as yet no confirmation from the Government of a date when this may be implemented.

The Health Visitor

The Health Visitor is a registered nurse (RGN) who has undertaken a special course at a College of Higher Education or university.

The workload of the Health Visitor is determined in two ways. Firstly, if she is attached to a G.P., she is responsible for the caseload of that practice even if this is scattered over a wide area. Secondly, if she is based in a geographical patch then she is responsible for clients within that defined area and may therefore liaise with many different G.P.s. Although most Health Visitors are attached to a G.P. there are local variations to cope with local needs. The Health Visitor determines who and when to visit and accepts referrals from many other agencies such as the school health service and social workers. In addition she may visit if she learns of a family or individual in need. For example a neighbour may be concerned about an elderly person becoming confused. Unlike most other social and health workers the Health Visitor provides a universal outreach service; that is she visits families on a regular basis without necessarily being asked to call. The pattern of visiting is based on individual family needs such as the birth of a new baby.

The Health Visitor is contacted at the local health centre or health clinic and families do frequently ask the Health Visitor to call, viewing her as a source of help for many social and health problems. However the Health Visitor also has an unique access to a wide range of families who are well and are therefore not seen routinely by other agencies such as social workers.

The Health Visitor sees all social classes and across all age ranges. Traditionally she is concerned with maternal and child health but her role has been widened to include all family members and groups such as the elderly and the handicapped. She goes to the families in their own homes and gives support and advice on all areas related to health and development. A major focus of her work is health education both to individuals and increasingly to groups such as mother and toddler, school children and women's health associations. There are many pressures on the health visiting service to further broaden the span of work because of the growing emphasis on health education and the recognition of the importance of prevention. Some pressures are the growing number of elderly people, the greater emphasis on shifting of care into the community for groups such as the mentally ill and mentally handicapped and the increase of family stress due to factors such as unemployment and family breakdown.

While the main focus of work is on home visiting, the Health Visitor is also responsible for child health clinics and child developmental clinics, and in some areas for the school nursing and well women clinics. The pattern of health visiting varies according to local health needs and size of caseloads.

Health Visitor caseloads have been traditionally described in terms of the number of infant health cards they hold (between 150–900) but increasingly this is changing and recognition is given to the work of the Health Visitor with other groups such as the elderly and with parents who have their first child (Barker, 1984). While the health visiting service is adapted to local needs and resources, the principles of health visiting remain constant. In 1977 the Council For the Education and Training Of Health Visitors identified four principles of health visiting in a report entitled 'An Investigation Into The Principles of Health Visiting' (1977).

- The search for health needs
- The stimulation of an awareness of health needs
- The influence on policies affecting health
- The facilitation of health-enhancing activities

Recently a working group has re-examined these four principles and found that the actual interventions may have changed but the basic principles underpinning health visiting practice are still relevant to today (HVA & UK Standing Conference on Health Visitor Education, 1992). These principles are very abstract so it is useful to look at the examples in Table 2.1.

Table 2.1   The principles of health visiting.

Principle	Examples
Search for health needs	Identifying health-damaging behaviour such as inadequate diet or unrecognised depression. Assessing community health needs.
Stimulation of the awareness of health needs	Encouraging individual to change health-damaging behaviour. Encouraging a local community to set up a group for isolated mothers.
Influence on policies affecting health	Identifying a group with particular health needs and presenting a case to nursing management for a change in service provision. This might be the establishment of a Well Women Clinic. Campaign for a change in housing provision.
Facilitation of health enhancing activities	Providing the means by which clients can be helped, e.g. setting up a stress reduction clinic or a series of health talks for teenagers.

The District Nurse

The District Nurse is an RGN who has undertaken post-basic training in a polytechnic (mandatory since 1981) to enable her to give skilled nursing care to all persons living outside hospital and to arrange financial and social help for them where appropriate. Within the

Primary Health Care Team (PHCT) she is the leader of the district nursing team.

As leader, the District Nurse delegates work to first and second level nurses and nursing auxiliaries or care assistants in her team but she remains wholly accountable for monitoring the care a patient receives. As you will have realised the District Nurse can be compared to a ward sister delegating work to her staff.

One-third of all nurses working in the community are District Nurses. They are usually very experienced – indeed 66% have been in their current job for over five years (Dunnell and Dobbs, 1982). The overwhelming majority (85%) are attached to a G.P. practice; however, the night and evening District Nurses often work a geographical patch. Attached District Nurses are responsible for the patients on one or more G.P.'s lists and patients are usually referred to them by the G.P. They also accept referrals from other members of the PHCT or directly from the hospital liaison sister who is often a community nurse.

Over the past few years District Nurses' case loads have increased in size and complexity. Some of the reasons for this are:

- Increasing numbers of elderly people
- The policy of a day surgery and early discharge for hospital patients which leads to a greater need for after-care and continuing rehabilitation in the community
- The increasing emphasis on care in the community for children, the mentally ill/handicapped, the physically disabled and the old
- Emphasis on home care for the terminally ill
- Increased public expectations of care
- Social and population changes (e.g. ethnic minorities, smaller families) all increase the need for support and health education in the community.

As shown in Fig. 2.4, the majority of the District Nurse's work is in the patients' home – though this may be an elderly or disabled persons' residential accommodation.

The District Nurse's key responsibilities are:

- Assessing and meeting the nursing needs of patients in the community.
- Applying skills and knowledge and imparting them effectively to patients, relatives, other carers and the general public (e.g. teaching safe lifting techniques or advising on the various financial benefits available).
- Communicating, establishing and maintaining good relationships and co-ordinating appropriate services for the patient, his family and others involved with delivery of care.
- Leading the district nursing team and understanding management and organisational principles within the multidisciplinary team.

- Promoting new developments to meet changing health care needs. (Adapted from the District Nurse Curriculum)

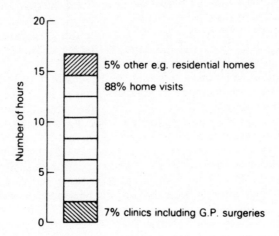

Fig. 2.4 District Nurse's work setting

District Nurses work predominantly with the elderly, chronically sick and the terminally ill. Their patients therefore are those whose problems 'defy precise definition, do not have readily available cures and are often prolonged' (Knopke and Diekelman, 1981).

She must ensure that her patients receive comprehensive and continuous care. Therefore she must take responsibility not only for district nursing care but also for liaising, co-ordinating and where appropriate delegating to other people.

One of the distinguishing features of community patients – as opposed to the hospital patient – is that they are usually 'on the books' for many years. The district nursing service is intermittent, providing in general only up to four visits in 24 hours. The District Nurse must therefore be skilled in what can be termed 'distanced' management. It is an important fact that even when the District Nurse is not physically present, she is responsible for the continuity of care provided. Indeed ultimately the standard of care received will depend more on her managerial, social and persuasive skills in relation to the patient, the carers and other members of the Primary Health Care Team than on her own nursing skills while in the patient's home.

District nurses are responsible for the standard of care they provide. Fig. 2.5 summarises these responsibilities. They work as independent practitioners although they are managerially accountable to their nursing officer at a Health Centre or District Office. As Charlotte Kratz put it:

District Nurses cannot usually be observed by their peers and their supervisors when at work: only by their patients and their patients' carers. This gives District Nurses tremendous independence. They can decide whom to visit and what to do when they get there. It also gives them tremendous responsibility. If they do not see or do something it will not be seen or done. If they are slipshod, negligent or callous in their work, only they and the patient will know and the patient may be unable or unwilling to complain.

(Barber and Kratz, 1980)

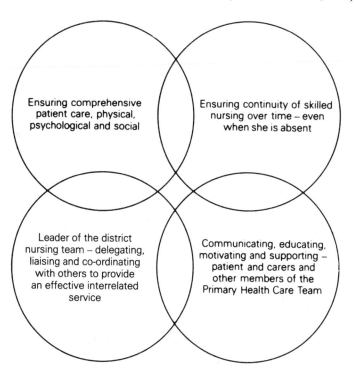

Fig. 2.5   The District Nurse's responsibilities

The Practice Nurse

Practice Nurses are employed by a general practitioner to work, as the name suggests, mainly in the G.P.'s surgery. In recent years there has been a dramatic increase in the numbers of Practice Nurses, this is due in no small part to the 1990 G.P. contract which has meant that Practice Nurses are not simply desirable but essential to achieve many of the targets within the contract. At the time of writing the training of all community nurses is under revue (community PREPP). It would seem that in future, instead of the present short certificate of attendance course, Practice Nurses will undergo an education programme that is equal to traditional post registrational community nursing education. This change is recognition that practice nursing is now an essential part of community nursing education.

The development of practice nursing

Practice nursing is not a new idea. Bowling and Stilwell (1988) noted that there were nurses working in general practice as early as 1910. However, practice nursing really started in 1965 following the implementation of the charter for the family doctor service which allowed 70% reimbursement of the cost of employing two ancillary staff for each practitioner. Although the majority of staff employed under this scheme were receptionists a few practice nurses were employed. In the mid 1970 to 1980s, the trend towards attaching Health Authority District Nurses to General Practitioners could have been expected to reduce the need for practice nurses, because a doctor could have a nurse for free, in fact there was a slight increase in the numbers of Practice Nurses. In 1975 the DHSS estimated that 650 whole time equivalent practice nurses were employed, whereas by 1982 there were 1000. Fig 2.6 shows the increase in the number of practice nurses between 1977 and 1989. It is apparent that there is a need for a Practice Nurse and that the role is different to that of the District Nurse or Health Visitor. As already mentioned, the 1990s has seen a rapid increase in both the numbers and the complexity of the role of the Practice Nurse. In the early days Practice Nurses functioned mainly as a receptionist and doctor's assistants, today's Practice Nurses are professionals in their own right and would be better described as collaborative practitioners rather than doctor's assistants.

What do Practice Nurses do? This is a difficult question to answer as the development of the role of the individual practice nurse is dependent on the need of the practice population, the employer's (G.P.) wishes, and the abilities and interest of the practice nurse.

The common activities that a Practice Nurse can carry out can be categorised under the following broad headings. The Practice Nurse you meet is unlikely to do all of the following.

- **Treatment Room Work**
  Dressing wounds, immunisation and vaccination clinics (for travellers, children, flu etc.), suturing, treating minor injuries and complaints, assisting with minor surgery, ear syringing, Venipuncture, ECGs etc. . .

- **Screening**
  Well person clinics, cervical cytology, hypertension and ischemic heart disease screening, elderly screening and human MOT etc. . .
- **Health Promotion**
  Both opportunistic or planned health promotion is carried out, such as placing posters and leaflets regarding healthy life style around the surgery. Lifestyle modification advice. Providing smoking, weight reduction, menopausal, retirement clinics and advice etc. . .
- **Management of Chronic Conditions**
  Monitoring health status, advising, teaching and supporting either on an individual basis or running designated clinic sessions for; diabetics, asthmatics, hypertensives etc. . .
- **Obstetrics and Family Planning**
  Assisting with ante- and post-natal care, Family planning etc. . .
- **Counselling**
  Providing information on services and opportunities open to patients, assisting patients come to terms with stressful situations etc. . .
- **Administration**
  Record keeping, nursing standards and protocol preparation, professional updating, research, input into purchasing contracts etc. . .

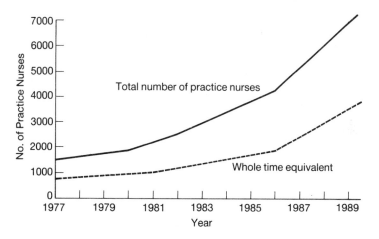

Fig. 2.6 Numbers of Practice Nurses 1977–1989 (Source: DHSS Figures)

Other nurses working in the community

Community Psychiatric Nurse (CPN)
Community Mental Handicap Nurse (CMHN)
Midwife
School nurse
Paediatric nurses

Elderly care teams
Diabetes nurse
Stoma nurses
Continence promotion nurses
Macmillan nurses
Oncology nurses

This book concentrates on the nurses you are most likely to spend your time with during your community placement, the District Nurse and the Health Visitor. There are many other nurses working in the community, most of which undertake a specialist rather than a generalist role, in that they work with specific client groups or medical conditions. They may be outreach workers from a hospital or based in the community. Most will serve a number of Primary Health Care Teams and they are an important and valued resource for nurses and patients in the community.

Student nurses undergoing pre-registration education will usually spend some time with the Community Midwife, Community Psychiatric Nurse (CPN), and/or the Community Mental Handicapped Nurse (CMHN) either in the common foundation programme or in the relevant branches.

Specialist nurses who work with particular client groups or medical conditions in the community give advance nursing care and act as consultants to generalist community nurses and the Primary Health Care Team as a whole. Diabetes nurses for example, can be a source of information to the District Nurse who is caring for the patients day to day needs.

Many specialist nurses work in the interphase between primary and secondary care, that is between community and hospital. They have an important role to play in facilitating the early discharge of patients from hospital, but perhaps more importantly, their expertise can reduce the need for many people to go into hospital in the first place.

Other members of the Primary Health Care Team

The Social Worker

In some areas the social worker is attached to a general practice in the same way as nurses but many social workers still work in a geographical area and liaise with many Primary Health Care Teams. In addition social workers work in many different settings such as hospitals, residential homes, children's homes and with voluntary agencies such as the National Society for the Prevention of Cruelty to Children.

In some areas social workers concentrate either upon a particular client group such as the handicapped, or upon different phases of work, such as work undertaken with local community development schemes.

The main client groups are the elderly, families in which there are neglected, abused or delinquent children, offenders, handicapped people and emotionally distressed people.

The role of the local authorities social service departments has changed following the 1990 NHS and Community Care Act from mainly providing services e.g. home helps and old peoples homes to the assembling and purchasing of 'packages' of care for their clients. In addition to this case management function, social workers provide help and support to the mentally ill and the care and protection of children. A large element of their work is with individuals and families who have severe social problems and need counselling and practical help.

The General Practitioner
Job Definition (Royal College of General Practitioners)

The General Practitioner is a doctor who provides personal, primary and continuing medical care to individuals and families. He may attend his patients in their homes, in his consulting-room or sometimes in hospital. He accepts the responsibility for making an initial decision on every problem his patients may present, consulting with specialists when he thinks it appropriate to do so. He will usually work in a group with other general practitioners, from premises that are built or modified for the purpose, with the help of paramedical colleagues, adequate secretarial staff and all the equipment which is necessary. Even if he is in single-handed practice, he will work in a team and delegate when necessary. His diagnoses will be composed in physical, psychological and social terms. He will intervene educationally, preventively and therapeutically to promote his patients' health.

Test yourself

1 What is a Primary Health Care Team?
2 Describe the roles of four members of a Primary Health Care Team.
3 What are the advantages of teamwork?

4   What is meant by Health Education?
5   What are the three levels of prevention?
6   Discuss the role of the different nurses in the team in relation to
    prevention.

3 The context in which Health Visitors work

Health Visitors are concerned with visiting a wide range of families across all social classes and age groups. As the Health Visitor sees families and individuals who are mainly well and functioning she is more concerned with needs than problems. As nursing students you may have been introduced to a problem solving approach and it can be difficult to understand working with people who are not ill or do not have an easily defined nursing problem.

The context of health visiting is different from what you may have experienced in hospital:

1   Health Visitors are often working with families and individuals who have *not* identified themselves as being in need of help.

2   Health Visitors *initiate* the majority of their visits so that they have to 'sell' themselves or take the lead in many of the visits.

3   Health Visitors have *long-term involvement* with families and communities. They often not only know the individual but also the family and social networks, knowledge which is often quite unique.

4   Health Visitors are often working with families in situations which are *difficult to change*. For example, many families are in poverty and very disadvantaged and there are few easy solutions to these problems.

5   Health Visitors have to work at the *pace of the individual* and family. For example, a woman who is a victim of violence may take some time to be able to leave home or even acknowledge the problem.

6   Health Visitors are concerned not with doing things *for* clients but are involved in doing things *with* the client.

7   Health Visitors are guests of the family; they are visiting families in their homes and *have no right of entry*.

8   Health Visitors are involved in working with the *community* and therefore have to liaise with community groups. This may involve group teaching or helping the community to identify and act on health problems. In this sense they work with people as a collective body and not only as individuals.

Although the Health Visitor uses knowledge from her nursing

background she tends not to be involved in practical nursing tasks such as dressings or giving injections. In this sense the skills used in health visiting are often difficult to appreciate when you first go out with her. The skills used are essentially social skills although there are some practical ones such as testing a baby's hearing.

In assessing the individual and the family from a social and health perspective the Health Visitor has to take many factors into consideration. She therefore has to build up a profile of the family over a number of visits, taking into account changing circumstances and the developing trust between herself and the family members. Often the families initially see the Health Visitor's work mainly focused on the baby and it may take some time for them to appreciate her wider role and knowledge. As a student you ought to be aware of the social factors which influence health such as poverty and encouraged to assess your client with these types of factors in mind. In order to confront the social factors influencing health daily, part of the Health Visitor's role is to work at a number of levels to improve health. Table 3.1 summarises the main skills used by a Health Visitor.

Firstly, the Health Visitor is concerned with helping individuals recognise health-damaging behaviour such as poor diet and motivate them to change that behaviour. This can be a very difficult and skilled task as any of you who have tried to give up smoking or to change eating habits will recognise. We may know something is bad for us but that does not necessarily mean we want to change our behaviour.

Secondly, she is involved in providing or encouraging others in the community to provide services or to start groups to meet health needs. This may involve the setting up of self-help groups for families with children with special needs or parents who have suffered bereavement from a sudden infant death. In addition the Health Visitor may have a contribution to make to local associations such as tenants or mother and toddler groups.

Thirdly, she tries to influence policies which affect health such as poor housing. This involves liaising with the local housing authorities to make her clients' need known. In addition Health Visitors can work through their professional organisations to bring these conditions to light.

Range of health visiting activities

The work of the Health Visitor varies throughout the United Kingdom in response to local need. For example, in inner city areas of London, Manchester and Edinburgh, they are working with homeless families who are living in hostels, hotels and boarding houses. In other areas of the country with a large number of elderly people, Health Visitors specialise in visiting this section of the population.

When you are working in the community it is necessary for you to ask how local need is being met by Health Visitors and what different patterns of work there are in your area. Despite local and innovatory schemes there are key activities which you could expect to see during your community experience.

Table 3.1 Main health visiting skills

Skill	Example
Teaching	explaining nutritional requirements demonstrating sterilization of feeding equipment
Questioning and reinforcing	assessing client needs
Advising	on immunisation schedules on social security benefits
Motivating/encouraging	the community to take up a health issue a client to attend for cervical cytology
Listening and supporting	in times of stress when there is a problem with no easy solution
Reflection of feeling and paraphrasing	when the client is bereaved when the client has a number of options to work through
Referral	to social services to voluntary agencies
Organisational	determining priorities in every caseload
Screening	hearing tests
Anticipatory guidance	to prepare parents for next stage of development
Monitoring/surveillance	child development
Advocacy	acting on behalf of, and with, the client or community in relation to other services such as the G.P. or the Supplementary Benefits Office

The young family antenatal to school age

Health Visitors maintain contact with clients on the basis of assessment of need and in negotiation with clients. Contact is maintained mainly through home visiting and by the provision of clinic sessions and group work.

The pattern of visits/contacts will vary from district to district and depend on individual family need, local community needs, caseload size and local policy. As child health surveillance forms an important part of the Health Visitors' work with pre-school children and their families, contact is often arranged to coincide with the requirements of the child health surveillance programme.

Since the minimum core programme for child health surveillance was proposed by the Joint Working Party on Child Health Surveillance (Hall, 1989, 1991) many G.P. practices and Health Authorities have implemented it and contact with families is arranged in accordance with the programme. Parental concern or professional judgement may mean that a child may be seen on more or different occasions from those listed in the visiting/contact guide. Bearing this in mind the visiting/contact pattern presented below is given as guidance only.

Visiting/contact guide

Antenatal visit on notification from G.P., midwife or hospital
Primary visit 10 to 14 days after birth
One or two visits/contacts in first six weeks
6/8 week examination
3 month visit/contact
6–9 months check
12 month visit/contact
18–24 months check
36 months–48 months pre-school examination

The objective of child health surveillance is to prevent disease, early detection of any problems which affect growth and development and to promote health. Health professionals work in collaboration with parents to achieve this objective. Child health surveillance is conducted through home visiting and through clinic work. Hearing and vision screening form part of child health surveillance.

Clinic work

In addition to home visiting Health Visitors see clients at Child Health Clinics and Well Baby Clinics. These clinics are attended by a community medical officer or G.P. for consultations, physical and developmental examinations and for immunisations. Mothers can have their babies weighed, meet other mothers and have access to health advice from Health Visitors. Subsidised baby milk and cheap vitamins are available.

In many districts there are paediatric developmental examination clinics where Health Visitors carry out a range of developmental checks including hearing and vision tests. The value of routine developmental examinations on all children has been questioned (Hall Report 1989, 1991) and in its place a new approach is proposed which places greater emphasis on parental observations in detecting developmental problems and greater reliance on professional judgement therefore replacing the need to carry out routine, detailed developmental examinations. In addition, the report proposes greater emphasis be placed on the health education aspect of the child health surveillance programme. Controversy surrounds the recommendations of the report and only time will tell whether as Robertson (1991, p90) states '. . . the proposed basic core programme and surrounding activities fare any better than the existing schemes, either in early discovery and/or as a basis for health education and support'.

In Health Centres and Health Clinics a range of other clinic sessions are provided in which Health Visitors may be involved. These include: well women clinics, family planning clinics, audiology sessions, ophthalmology clinics, elderly screening clinics, child guidance clinics.

School health services

In some areas there are school nurses who are totally responsible for the school health services, while in others the Health Visitor has considerable involvement. The school health service offers:

1   Medical inspections, including booster immunisation, vision and hearing testing in the first year in primary school.
2   Health inspection at 7 years of age including colour, vision and hearing. A medical examination may be conducted if deemed necessary.
3   Rubella immunisation at 11 years of age for girls and BCG testing and vaccination for all children at 13 years of age.
4   Follow-up health checks for children with special problems such

as enuresis.
5   Liaison work between school and home about children with a
range of social and health problems.
6   A range of health education sessions throughout the age ranges,
covering personal health needs from dental health to preparation for
parenthood. This may be undertaken in conjunction with teachers as
part of the personal and social development element of the national
curriculum.

In many areas the Health Visitor links the school to the community
and encourages community projects of relevance to elderly people
and people with special needs.

Liaison activities

Health Visitors, because they are visiting a wide range of the population who are not in contact with other health and social services, can
identify people in need and are identified as being in a key position
for liaison work, including:

- Identifying women with social and health problems at antenatal
  clinics
- Following up antenatal defaulters
- Home reports preceding discharge for premature babies, children
  and elderly people
- Home conditions and social reports for children in paediatric
  wards
- Follow-up visits for cervical cytology
- Linking with social workers, NSPCC, G.P.s in child protection
  cases
- Links with voluntary agencies such as Women's Aid or Mencap
- Follow-up of infectious diseases such as TB or contacting venereal
  disease cases
- Linking with the local DSS office in response to claimants'
  requests
- Linking with local services such as housing, public health or
  social services
- Linking with local hospital such as psychiatric or general

Group health education

This is an increasing area of the Health Visitor's work and
includes: health promotion associations such as 'stop smoking'

groups, parentcraft classes in hospital or clinic, school children and teenagers, groups for elderly people, mother and toddler groups, women's health groups, groups with special needs such as parents with children with special needs or parents who have a sudden infant death, young adolescent groups, various local groups such as Tenants Groups or Workers' Education Association, and outreach schemes such as radio phone-in services or stalls in local markets.

Specialisation

Although the health visiting service is said to be generic there are some Health Visitors who work in specialised areas. These include: working with elderly people, minority ethnic groups, children with special needs, homeless families, case finding for special clinics and abusing parents.

Test yourself

1 What is the core programme of Child Health Surveillance?
2 What group health education sessions are being undertaken by the Health Visitor?
3 Who comes to the child health clinic?
4 What links has the Health Visitor with the local schools?
5 How much involvement does the Health Visitor have with the elderly population in the area?

4   The Health Visitor and family assessment

Health Visitors are involved in assessing health needs, planning, implementing and evaluating health visiting – activities which are similar to the nursing process.

Assessment

The emphasis is not solely problem-centred but must involve looking at actual and potential need. Health Visitors are also concerned with identifying resources which are available to the individual and group, e.g. in social networks, the local community or from within the person themselves.

The next stage is to assist the client to articulate their own needs, and to establish if these needs are recognised by the rest of the family.

The final stage is to make sense of this range of information in order to compile an assessment which adequately represents the needs, problems and resources of the individual (Orr, 1985).

When the Health Visitor has assessed the individual or family it is often the case that there are a range of outcomes for each case:

1   No need exists, the individual is well and will be reassessed at specific intervals linked to developmental stages, for example, or to life change events such as the birth of a child.
2   No need exists but a potential need may be offset, for example, by giving information. This is the primary prevention stage.
3   A need exists but is being handled successfully by individual, or other agencies and periodic reassessment will be planned.
4   A need exists and the individual requires help in handling it. This help may be the giving of information, providing support or counselling, obtaining resources or referral to other agencies.
5   A need exists which the client cannot handle and does not recognise and intervention is required for a short time. An example of this might be the need for nutritional advice. This is the secondary stage of prevention.

6 A need exists which must be monitored over a long period of time, for example, when a child seems to be slow in reaching developmental milestones.

7 A need is imposed unexpectedly upon the individual and crisis intervention is required, as in the case of sudden homelessness or a severe home accident.

8 A need is long-term and permanent and for which the individual requires some continuous, intermittent or initial help. An example of such tertiary prevention is the existence of a chronic handicapping condition.

Planning health visiting interventions in conjunction with clients involves:

- Assigning priorities to the recognised needs
- Deciding which needs could be resolved: without assistance or with the aid of social networks, by other agencies such as social workers or by the Health Visitor herself
- Designating specific actions to immediate, medium term and long term goals
- Recording needs, actions and expected outcomes

Implementation

This phase involves putting the plan into action, initiating and completing strategies which will lead to the achievement of defined goals.

The final stage of evaluation involves the measuring of outcomes against the stated goals.

Family and individual assessment

Health Visitors visit many families in which there are few problems. There may, however, be a need for information on a range of issues which affect health such as feeding, contraception or immunisation.

As a student nurse it may be difficult to understand the function of health visiting to families who are healthy and functioning. We should look at the practice of health visiting, the possible outcomes of a visit and what level of prevention exists. Let us first look at family assessment.

Despite the many variations of families and individuals with which the Health Visitor works there are certain factors which are taken into account when an assessment is being made. These are summarised in Fig. 4.1. As you read the following case studies bear these factors in mind.

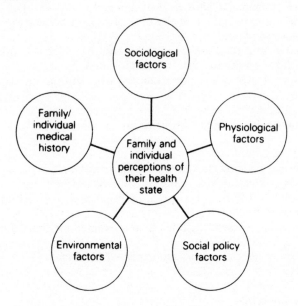

Fig. 4.1   Factors in a health visiting assessment

Factors in health visiting assessment of any family

Individual and family details: the Health Visitor is assessing if the family members are healthy and what potential problems there may be. It is important therefore to look at the type of family in terms of sex, age, relations within the family and racial or religious background. For example it would be important to know the dietary beliefs of an Asian family before discussing nutrition.

Medical history: It is also important to know what illnesses or injuries the various family members have had in the past as well as their current state of health. For example there are diseases such as diabetes which may affect the outcome of a pregnancy.

Environmental factors: the health of the family will be affected by the type of housing and the area in which they live. If, for example, the family have poor housing and live in a deprived area they may have inadequate heating or the children may have no place to play and be at risk of street accidents.

Sociological factors: family health is affected by the level of income and this is largely dependent on the educational level of family members and what jobs they have and on the economic climate. It is obvious in our society that some occupations have more status than others and provide a higher standard of living. For example there is a noteable difference between the life style of a hospital consultant and a hospital porter and this is reflected nationally in the different levels of mortality and morbidity with those in the professional and managerial professions having fewer illnesses and a longer life expectancy ('Black Report', DHSS 1982). The beliefs that people hold about the causes of ill health are also linked to educational level and status. It is often the case that semi-skilled and unskilled workers do not use preventive health services such as cervical screening as much as other groups. Because of low income and lack of knowledge they may be unable to adopt life styles which lead to good health e.g. having an adequate diet. We are influenced in health matters not only by our immediate family but also by the extended family of grandparents, etc. We need to know therefore to what extent the mother of a new baby, for example, is influenced by the advice given by her sisters, etc.

Psychological factors: There is an increasing recognition that ill health is related to social and emotional stress. The Health Visitor therefore has to be aware of how the family is coping with stressful life events such as the birth of a new baby or changes in housing or jobs. Because the Health Visitor works mainly with women she is concerned with the way women see themselves and how much control they have over their lives. The woman's level of self-esteem, for example, is related to the quality of the environment that she will be able to provide for her children in terms of helping their development.

Social policy factors: a wide range of health and welfare services are available to families and it is the job of the Health Visitor to ensure that families know about these services as well as the relevant social security benefits.

At the centre of any family assessment is how the family members define their own health problems and needs and also to what extent they are able to deal with these themselves, obtain help from friends and relatives, or use health and welfare services. Within a health visiting assessment for a family there is an individual assessment covering the major body systems and factors which may lead to ill health.

Individual health assessment

- General health and mood
- Specific problems: rashes, pains
- Past medical history: operations, long-term conditions
- Family medical history: diabetes
- Medications: contraceptive pill, indigestion tablets

- Allergies
- Life style: exercise, occupation and work hazards, rest, nutrition
- Health-damaging behaviours: smoking, alcohol
- Gastrointestinal system: constipation, dental health
- Urogenital systems: cystitis, vaginal health, pre-menstrual tension
- Respiratory system: persistent cough
- Infections: flu

Let us now look at the work of the Health Visitor with an antenatal family, a family with young children and an elderly woman living alone.

The role of Health Visitors in antenatal visiting

The Health Visitor has a major health education role in the antenatal period both in parentcraft classes and in home visiting. Ideally contact would be made as early in pregnancy as possible as it facilitates the development of a working relationship with the client, provides the opportunity to explain about the health visiting service and to offer health education. This visit may need to be in the evening to accommodate working women and to have the opportunity to meet with fathers. Competing caseload pressures may mean that Health Visitors are unable to visit all antenatal clients and therefore the service has to be targeted at those women who are most in need. This would include primiparous mothers who have been shown to experience greater anxiety in the antenatal and early post-natal period than multiparous mothers (Snelson *et al.*, 1990). Women with a poor obstetric history and women whose social circumstances may put them in greater need, e.g. women living in poverty, in poor housing or who are homeless would also be priority cases. Health Visitors should be able to identify women who are at special risk and put them in touch with the health and social services as early as possible.

There is a move to reach women planning to have children before conception occurs so that they can be offered health advice regarding an adequate diet, avoiding drugs, smoking and alcohol, and have their immune status checked for infections such as rubella, toxoplasmosis which if caught during pregnancy can seriously affect the health of the fetus. In some areas there are pre-conceptual clinics or this service may be offered at some well women clinics but for most women they only receive the relevant health advice when they become pregnant. In all cases, however, the care of the pregnant woman should begin as early as possible according to the Short Report (1980) and the DHSS (1977) in Prevention and Health: Reducing the Risk.

Examples of health education topics relevant during the antenatal period:

- Physical changes
- Rest and exercise
- Environmental dangers such as X-rays, passive smoking, toxoplasmosis, listeria and anticipatory guidance regarding home safety
- Dental health
- Sexual changes
- Emotional changes and acceptance of role changes
- Preparation for birth and the immediate post-natal period, encouragement of breastfeeding
- Lifestyle including smoking, alcohol, drugs and nutrition, financial benefits and services available.

Lifestyle – why it is important

> Evidence suggests that persuading mothers not to smoke cigarettes would do more to reduce infant mortality in the UK than any other single action.
>
> *DHSS in Prevention and Health* (1977)

Smoking. Mothers who smoke increase the possibility of having 'small for date' babies. There is also a high incidence of premature babies, an increased risk of spontaneous abortion and smokers also suffer poorer health themselves. In addition, there is increasing evidence of the dangers of passive smoking for both the mother, her unborn child and other children in the household. Passive smoking has been shown to cause lung cancer in nonsmokers and serious respiratory illness in babies (e.g. bronchitis, pneumonia). It is also associated with an increased risk of developing heart disease, with chronic middle ear disease in children, and with aggravating asthma. There is also some evidence to suggest a link between passive smoking and birth weight. Babies born to mothers who have been exposed to passive smoking tend to weigh less than babies born to unexposed mothers (Froggatt Report, 1988). Low birth weight babies are more susceptible to infection and developing complications post-natally.

Alcohol affects the mother's digestive system and reduces the absorption of a number of nutrients including Vitamin A, Vitamin C, folic acid, iron and zinc.

Even small amounts of alcohol affect the fetus and in excess can cause Fetal Alcohol Syndrome. This means that a baby may have craniofacial abnormalities, retarded growth, nervous system damage (e.g. mental handicap) or physical abnormalities.

Nutrition. A mother's nutritional status on entering pregnancy has a significant influence on birth weight and neonatal outcome.

The importance of dietary advice pre-conceptually can not be over emphasised. Following the diagnosis of pregnancy improving the diet may improve the mother's health and the quality of breast milk but only has a modest effect on birth size (Doyle *et al.*, 1991). An assessment of a pregnant woman's diet should focus as much on the quality of the diet as on the quantity. As long as weight gain during pregnancy remains within normal limits (3.5–4 kg by the end of 20 weeks of pregnancy and thereafter just under 0.5 kg per week until term) it may be assumed that energy intake is adequate. Pregnancy and lactation increases nutrient requirements in particular for folic acid, iron, calcium and zinc.

Examples of sources rich in these nutrients include:

- **Folic acid**   whole grain cereals, eggs and wholemeal bread, sweet potato
- **Iron**   red meat, liver, cereals, dark green vegetables and pulses (e.g. chick peas, blackeyed beans)
- **Calcium**   milk (skimmed and semi-skimmed), yoghurt, cheese, sardines and tofu
- **Zinc**   red meat, liver, wholegrain cereals, cheese

Any dietary advice offered must be tailored to the individual's needs and take into account cultural and personal beliefs and values as well as being within the individual's financial means.

Case history

Miss Sarah Green and Mr Bob Harris have been co-habiting for one year in a privately rented one bedroom flat in an inner city area. Miss Green is 20 years old and is seven months pregnant with her first child. She has just stopped working as a shop assistant. She does not smoke and only drinks 'at Christmas and on special occasions'. Miss Green's mother lives nearby but she cares for her two younger children aged 14 and 12 as well as caring for her elderly mother who sustained a stroke six months ago. Miss Green's father works as a hospital porter.

Mr Harris is 24 years old and works nights on a car production line. Due to the recession the company has recently announced the need to cut jobs at the plant. It is hoped that this can be achieved through voluntary redundancy but the future looks pessimistic and morale is low at the plant. Mr Harris's father also works at the plant, whilst his mother works part-time as a school cleaner as well as minding her young grandson for her other son and daughter-in-law.

The Health Visitor was notified of Miss Green's pregnancy from the large maternity hospital where she is attending for antenatal care.

The Health Visitor contacted Miss Green to arrange a convenient time to visit. As Mr Harris works nights a late afternoon visit was chosen so that both parents could have the opportunity to meet the Health Visitor.

Whilst the Health Visitor may have several aims for the visit it is essential that she finds out from the family what they see as their needs and ensures that these are addressed before pursuing any aims she may have for the visit. In this way each antenatal visit is unique, tailored to the needs of a particular family. The aims listed below are therefore offered as guidance only.

Health visiting aims for an antenatal visit:

1   To introduce yourself to the couple and to begin to develop a working relationship
2   To explain the role of the Health Visitor
3   To find out and discuss any concerns which the couple have
4   To enquire about the preparations the couple have made for the arrival of their first baby and to help prepare them for the event
5   To assess the couple's physical, emotional and social health
6   To offer health advice on nutrition, smoking, dental health, exercise/rest, sex in pregnancy, home safety and emotional changes
7   To discuss with the couple their expectations of parenthood
8   To discuss the chosen method of infant feeding
9   To inform the couple of available financial benefits and services

Miss Green warmly welcomed the Health Visitor in, offered her a cup of tea and asked that she call them Sarah and Bob. Bob poked his head around the door, said 'Hello' and offered to make the tea. The flat was warm and comfortable. Sarah said they were lucky to have a good landlord who ensured the flat is well maintained, although the rent is high. At this early stage in the visit the Health Visitor did not feel it was appropriate to discuss finances but would hope to pursue this later in the visit if it was again raised by Sarah.

The Health Visitor explained that she had come to answer any questions the couple may have, to inform them of services available in the area and of the Health Visitor's role before and after the birth. Bob brought in the tea and was about to leave when the Health Visitor explained that she had come to see both of them. Bob was a little surprised as he thought that Health Visitors were only for mothers and young children, but willingly sat down and became involved in the discussion. The Health Visitor asked 'How's the pregnancy going?' – an open-ended question to get the couple talking.

Sarah stated that she regularly attended the antenatal clinic, that she was gaining weight appropriately and that all was progressing well. She stated that she was having to take iron supplements and that this was making her constipated. This provided an opportunity to discuss diet with Sarah. She recounted what she had eaten the day before which contained a wide range of foods including cereal and white bread, fruit and vegetables, red meat, tuna fish, tea and coffee with no sugar and skimmed milk. The Health Visitor asked whether this was a typical day's menu and then praised Sarah on her balanced diet. To help the constipation, Sarah was advised to increase her fluid and fibre intake. This could be achieved by changing to wholemeal bread and to a bran-based cereal, and by increasing her consumption of milk, fruit juices and water whilst limiting her tea and coffee intake. The Health Visitor explained that having fruit juice with a meal increased the absorption of iron as it was a rich source of Vitamin C whilst tea and coffee inhibited it. A fluid intake of approximately 7 glasses per day should be adequate. Sarah was very interested in her diet and seemed keen to take up the Health Visitor's advice, although felt that limiting her tea and coffee intake would be hard. Bob commented that he also liked his coffee with two sugars! This led into a discussion about dental health. Sarah explained that she was having her teeth checked next week whilst it was free. She was informed that she was eligible to receive free dental treatment up until the baby is one year old. The Health Visitor asked Bob whether he attended the dentist regularly and he stated that he had not been since he was a child. She said he disliked dentists and even though he had toothache he would not go. 'When the pain gets really bad then I'll have to go but I'm not going until then.' The Health Visitor accepted Bob's decision and discussed home remedies which may ease his toothache and the possibility of reducing his sugar intake to prevent further dental decay. A Health Visitor can not tell people what to do, only ensure that they have been offered all the information to enable them to make an informed decision. Bob is fully aware of the benefits of preventive dental care and dental treatment but chooses at the moment not to take advantage of the service.

The conversation then turned to the couple's expectations of parenthood. The reality of parenthood can be far removed from the glowing photographs of contented babies in magazines. Sarah explained that the pregnancy was unplanned and initially had come as quite a shock. However, over the months they had become used to the idea and were looking forward to the birth. 'Well' Sarah said 'not the labour, but having the baby'. She admitted to feeling anxious about the labour and asked about the availability of pain relief. The Health Visitor reassured her that it was natural to feel anxious and then went on to explain about labour and various methods of pain relief. This topic amongst others will be covered at the parentcraft classes which Sarah is planning to attend. Bob hopes to be able to attend some of the sessions especially the session on labour as he intends to be present at the birth. Sarah is keen to meet other pregnant women in the area as she is already missing her work colleagues. The Health Visitor then gives them a copy of 'Birth to Five', a Health Education Authority (1989) publication which provides useful information on pregnancy, baby care and the first five years of the child's life. This booklet is full of helpful health advice which the couple can read at their leisure and refer to when appropriate.

The Health Visitor then steers the conversation on to a new topic by asking 'Have you decided on how you are going to feed the baby?' 'Well I think I will probably bottle feed. I know breast is best and all that but I was bottle fed and Bob was too and he says he will help me with the feeds if I bottle feed so I think I've made my mind up really'. Research evidence (Hally *et al*, 1981) shows that the method of infant feeding is decided very early on in pregnancy re-emphasising the need for more pre-conceptual care and increased health education with school children about breastfeeding. The partner is very influential in the decision to breastfeed or not. If the partner is not supportive of breastfeeding the mother is less likely to succeed or even attempt breastfeeding (Hally *et al.*, 1981; Solberg, 1985). Once the decision has been made it is important that the Health Visitor supports the couple in their decision and ensures that they are offered all the information necessary to successfully and safely bottle feed.

The Health Visitor then inquires about arrangements the couple have made for after the baby is born. Sarah reports that Bob has arranged to take a week's holiday when she comes home from hospital and that her mother and mother-in-law will help as far as they are able. Sarah reports that she is concerned about her mother and that 'She looks dreadful. She's tired all the time and her back's causing her trouble but she says she hasn't the time to go to the doctors. Gran can be very demanding'. The Health Visitor offers to call round to her mother's who is also registered with the same G.P. to assess her mother's health and to ensure she is receiving all the services and benefits to which she is entitled to help her care for her elderly mother. Sarah seems relieved by this and goes on to explain that everyone at the moment is feeling stressed. Bob lights a cigarette and talks about the job cuts at work and his fears for the future. 'I don't know how we would manage if I lost my job. We haven't any savings or anything and my Dad might be laid off too.' The Health Visitor makes a mental note of the need to discuss Bob's smoking with the couple when she next sees them. It is inappropriate to discuss it now as it is a particularly stressful time for Bob and smoking may be his coping strategy for dealing with the stress. Instead she informs them of the maternity benefits to which they are entitled and child benefit following the baby's birth. She also informs them of Social

Security benefits which would be available in the event that Bob lost his job and that the Citizen Advice Bureau or welfare rights office were excellent sources of advice regarding benefits available and employment rights. This led on to a discussion about other services and benefits available.

Services and Benefits for Antenatal Women

- Antenatal clinics at hospital or shared care with G.P. and midwife
- Parentcraft classes and relaxation classes at hospital or local clinic
- Free dental care, glasses, prescriptions, chiropody
- Midwives
- Health Visitors
- Cheap vitamins available at child health clinic
- Financial benefits
  Statutory Maternity Pay (SMP) – paid by employer. The amount depends on length of time in present employment.
  Maternity Allowance – for pregnant women who have recently given up a job or who work but are not eligible for SMP. The allowance is payable for 18 weeks.
  Maternity Expenses Payment – for pregnant women who are or their partners are in receipt of Income Support, Family Credit or Disability Working Allowance. This is a means-tested benefit to assist with buying equipment and items for the baby. It can be claimed up until the baby is three months old. [DSS leaflets *Babies and Benefits* (FB8), *Maternity Benefits* (NI/7A) and *A Guide to the Social Fund* (SB16) provide detailed information and are available from any DSS office or post office.]

The visit had already lasted an hour and the Health Visitor was conscious that a lot of information had been exchanged. She asked them whether there was anything else they wanted to ask, before summarising the main points, reminding the couple about the parentcraft classes and leaving them a contact number where they could reach her.

It must be remembered that health visiting is a long term activity and that the Health Visitor will be in regular contact with this family in the early post-natal period and will maintain contact until the child goes to school. This provides the opportunity to review health needs identified at this visit and to offer health advice and anticipatory guidance as and when appropriate. Following this visit the Health Visitor identifies the couple's health needs as:

1 Stress resulting from threatened job loss and limited finances
2 Stress over the health of Sarah's mother
3 Bob's smoking and the danger of passive smoking for Sarah and the baby
4 Bob's dental health

5   Sarah's constipation
6   A social need for Sarah to meet other pregnant women in the area.

These needs will be reviewed when the Health Visitor next sees the couple at the parentcraft classes.

Test yourself

1   What antenatal services exist in the area in which you work?
2   What topics are covered in the parentcraft classes at your clinic?
3   What happens when a pregnant woman 'books in' at the local midwifery hospital?
4   How often and at what stage in the pregnancy do Health Visitors visit in the antenatal period?
6   What skills does the Health Visitor have in visiting antenatal women and what topics are covered?

The family with young children

When you are in the community you will see the Health Visitor mainly visiting families with children under 5 years of age. As in the antenatal period, her main role will be one of prevention, health promotion and monitoring the health needs of all the family members. She works mainly with women and children although in areas of high male unemployment she may be meeting more fathers.

Case history

The Taylor family lives in a semi-detached house in a suburb of a large town. Mr. Taylor is 34 years old and is employed as a computer programmer. Mrs Taylor is 32 and worked as a teacher before the birth of her first child, Jane, three years ago. Her second child, Mark, was born 14 days ago and the Health Visitor is due on a 'primary visit'. By this we mean the first visit following the birth of a new baby.

At this time, the Health Visitor is concerned with the health of the mother and baby and in assessing how the rest of the family have adapted to the change in family structure. Ideally, she will have met Mrs Taylor in the antenatal period. The Health Visitor will have been notified of the birth through the health authorities and will have received a child health record card. This card is to be completed and held by the Health Visitor until the child goes to school; then it is transferred to the school health service. If the family leaves the area, their records will be transferred. There are many details on this card, which form part of the Health Visitor's assessment (for example, the age of the mother and details of the birth). In many areas parent-held records have been introduced. The Health Visitor completes the record in the presence of the parents and they are encouraged to bring the record whenever they attend health services for the child. Parents are encouraged to write in the record and the record contains a wealth of useful health advice. A national child health record was launched in 1990. However, many areas have devised their own record to meet the needs of their particular communities. In some areas the parent-held record is the main record held, in others duplicate records are kept by the Health Visitor. The purpose of the parent-held record is to foster greater parental involvement and promote partnership between professionals and parents in the child's care.

In the case of the Taylor family, the Health Visitor will be assessing how 3 year old Jane is responding to the new baby and whether there is any jealousy. The possibility of sibling jealousy should have been discussed at an antenatal visit.

Primary visit – The baby

Examination of the baby:
1 Observe baby's general condition, colour and muscle tone;
2 Working from head to toes, check sutures, fontanelles, eyes, nose, mouth, skin folds, breasts, umbilicus, fingers, toes, genital areas, hips and check for presence of primitive reflexes – grasp, stepping and moro. The Health Visitor is looking for any abnormalities which may be present (e.g. cleft palate, torticollis, talipes, imperforate anus).

Feeding: The Health Visitor asks about the type of feeding, whether it is breast or bottle and if there are any difficulties in the baby sucking.

Often mothers who breast feed are concerned as to whether the baby is receiving an adequate intake of milk. The Health Visitor will enquire about and look for signs of an adequate intake including frequent wet nappies, stools of normal colour and consistency, sleeping between feeds, pink mucous membranes and weight gain of 142g to 225g per week (Talbot, 1989). If the baby is bottle fed, it is important to check on how the feed is made up and whether correct amounts of powder to water are used. Mothers can often add an extra scoop 'for luck'. Some mothers may have difficulty reading or understanding the instructions on the tin. The nature of sterilising the bottles is also important and general points about this may need repeating. It is often a good idea, if possible, to see the mother feed her baby and in this way to see how the baby is handled, how well it sucks and the relationship between the mother and child.

Warmth and safety: babies should be kept in temperatures of 65°F (18°C) and inexperienced mothers are often unsure about the correct amount of clothing and blankets. Babies can lose considerable heat from their heads and have difficulty generating heat so that they need to be placed in a cot which is already warmed. Most of the baby equipment is tested for safety but mothers need to be alerted to dangers from some carry cots, pillows, etc. If there are animals in the house, then a cat net should be used and hygiene precautions taken to prevent dogs licking babies or placing their dishes near baby feeding equipment.

Crying and irritability: the Health Visitor asks about the baby's pattern of sleeping, waking and crying, looking for any sign that there is excessive crying which is distressing for the baby and upsetting the parents. Babies tend to cry more than most parents expect and this can be a cause of great concern and stress. Parents need to check all the possible reasons for crying, e.g. thirst, hunger or discomfort, and learn to recognise the different type of cries which babies have.

Screening tests: the Health Visitor carries out a test for phenylketonuria and for hypothyroidism. Both of these disorders affect the baby's growth and mental development if left untreated. However, if detected early and appropriate treatment is commenced, the baby grows and develops normally. The baby's heel is pricked and a blood sample is placed on a specially treated card which is sent to the local hospital laboratory.

While the main focus of the visit so far is on the baby, the Health Visitor is assessing the mother and how she relates to and handles the baby. One of the main aims of this primary visit is to determine the mother's physical and emotional state, to enable her to talk about the experience of the birth and to discuss how she is adapting to motherhood. To accomplish this, the Health Visitor might ask such questions as:

- 'In the first hour after birth, how many minutes was the baby with you?'
- 'Did you feel that you were in control of what happened to you during the birth of your baby?'
- 'Did the midwives and doctors ask your opinion about how you wanted to have the baby, e.g. what position and pain relief?'

These types of questions will help Mrs Taylor to express her feelings. This is very important because there is growing evidence that many women are dissatisfied with the maternity care they received and need to work through any feelings of disappointment or anger (Oakley, 1979; Smith, 1989). The Health Visitor is aware that some mothers suffer from post-natal depression and in order to ascertain Mrs Taylor's mood she might ask:

- 'How well do you feel in yourself?'
- 'Do you feel tired most of the time?'
- 'Do you feel miserable or depressed?'

There are other stresses which may be causing the mother concern and the Health Visitor should ascertain whom Mrs Taylor can confide in and what help and support is available from friends and relatives. Many mothers find caring for a new baby very tiring and this may be especially the case when there is a 3 year old child as well. The Health Visitor should spend time encouraging Mrs Taylor to take care of herself, get as much rest as possible and eat a healthy diet with plenty of fluids, especially as she is breast feeding. She drinks milk and is taking additional iron as her haemoglobin was low in hospital. Fibre is encouraged to prevent constipation.

Many mothers expect too much of themselves and want to maintain the standards of housekeeping and commitment to the family they had before the baby was born. Mrs Taylor is very houseproud and feels that she should not let this slip. The Health Visitor explains that this is adding an extra strain to what is a considerable amount of work in caring for a new baby and toddler.

She suggests ways of cutting down the work by, for example, disposable nappies and asking Mr Taylor to help.

Mrs Taylor, although she feels tired, seems to be relaxed and confident in handling the baby. She is aware of the jealousy which Jane feels towards the baby and involves her as much as possible in the care of the baby, but sets time aside to spend alone with her. All visitors to the house are encouraged to make a special fuss of Jane and not go immediately to see the new baby.

Mrs Taylor is encouraged to attend for her postnatal check-up and to make an appointment with her G.P. She is following her postnatal exercises and her lochia is satisfactory. Her perineum is still tender as she had an episiotomy, but it is not giving her too much discomfort. The Health Visitor discusses family planning with Mrs Taylor. As she is breastfeeding she is taking the mini pill and is fully aware of the need for accuracy in the timing of taking it. Mrs Taylor is invited to the baby clinic and informed of the immunisation schedule and the child health surveillance programme.

Immunisation Schedule

2 months
Diphtheria
Tetanus
Pertussis
Oral Poliovaccine
Haemophilus Influenza Type B

3 months
Diphtheria
Tetanus
Pertussis
Oral Poliovaccine
Haemophilus Influenza Type B

4 months
Diphtheria
Tetanus
Pertussis
Oral Poliovaccine
Haemophilus Influenza Type B

12–18 months
Measles
Mumps
Rubella
(MMR)

4–5 years
Booster Diphtheria and Tetanus
Oral Poliovaccine

The Health Visitor is also concerned with Jane's development and in particular, with how she has adjusted to the arrival of a new baby. This often incites regressive behaviour with a return to bed wetting or temper tantrums to get attention because of confusion and anger at no longer being the centre of attention. In the antenatal period the Health Visitor will have discussed sibling jealousy and Mrs Taylor has been very anxious to avoid this and is managing to help Jane adjust.

Health Visitor has been encouraging Mrs Taylor to stimulate Jane and has tried to show her how to provide environmental opportunities within which development can take place. The structuring of the environment to help the child achieve various goals is something which applies throughout the early years, from the correct positioning and frequent changing of home-made mobiles in the earliest months, to the 'near-solution' of a jigsaw puzzle for the older toddler (so that an unpractised child has only one or two moves left to complete the puzzle). On the other hand the mother is advised not to create problem solving situations which are clearly well ahead of the child's present development level.

The Health Visitor helps Mrs Taylor to realise that Jane's mental abilities can be profoundly altered by the kinds of activities she is given – altered for the worse or for the better. At every age, it is possible to think up simple puzzle activities or 'problem-solving' tasks which will stimulate the child's imagination and mental functioning. It is preferable to leave only a small number of educational or other toys with Jane at any one time, to foster the child's powers of concentration.

There is a great deal that the Taylors can do to prepare Jane for school, right from the first year. The parents help particularly by showing her picture books and talking about the pictures, by reading stories to her every night before she goes to sleep, by playing simple number games and by teaching the child how to manipulate objects – for example, by sorting toys (into soft/hard, or other divisions), clothing (sizes or who they belong to) and eating utensils. In addition, Jane has been attending a mother and toddler group since the age of 18 months and will start a playgroup at the start of the new term. Playgroups provide excellent preparation for school, enabling the child to mix with children of their own age, to adapt to being separated from their mother and to interact with other adults. Figure 4.2 shows some of the different aspects involved in health assessments.

The Health Visitor will be assessing a range of developmental factors; as an example let us examine how Jane may be assessed on social and cognitive developments.

Social development

Is Jane able to:

- fetch named things
- copy Mother doing household work
- treat doll or teddy like a real child
- partly or fully dress herself
- comfort other children when they cry
- recognise that some things belong to others
- join in jokes and laughter with others
- clean her own teeth with help for the back teeth
- show new skills to strangers
- be willing to share toys
- play co-operatively with other children
- play on her own in games of imagination
- do house tasks to help family

Cognitive development

Is Jane able to:

- fetch a chair to reach something
- assemble a jigsaw
- sort things into similar groups
- pair things with other things
- find missing parts of a picture
- find the odd one out
- draw an 'egg' person
- draw a human figure
- aware of time periods
- aware of days of the week

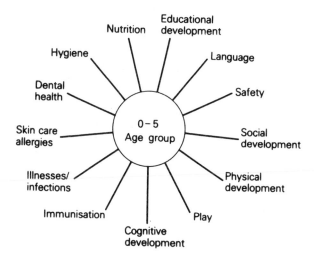

Fig. 4.2 Health assessment of young children

Health visiting and elderly people

To date, the work of Health Visitors with elderly people is an underdeveloped area. Yet, as demographic trends indicate a rising number of elderly people, especially those aged 85 years and over (OPCS, 1989), Health Visitors need to review their current practice of working predominantly with the 0–5 age group. Currently, contact with elderly people often occurs once a crisis has arisen. Whilst contact at this stage does enable the Health Visitor to offer health advice, to prevent problems occurring in the first place contact needs to be made much earlier.

The Health Visitor's role with elderly people consists of providing health education, screening and supportive care. The aim is to enable elderly people to live independently within the community for as long as possible by ensuring that they are receiving all relevant services and benefits.

It must be remembered that elderly people are not a homogenous group. This group will consist of individuals who may vary in age by up to thirty years or more, whose life experiences and medical histories are vastly different and whose needs are accordingly diverse. A detailed assessment of the individual's needs must be undertaken to ensure that these needs are addressed. Health education topics listed below which may be discussed with elderly clients are therefore offered as guidance only.

Examples of health education topics relevant for visiting elderly people include:

- safety – personal, home and road safety
- heating and preventing hypothermia
- nutritional advice
- immunisation, e.g. influenza, tetanus
- foot care
- exercise in later life
- services, self-help groups (e.g. carers groups) and financial benefits available

Health education may be offered on a one to one basis during a home visit or through group work, e.g. pre-retirement groups, carers groups, etc.

To facilitate making early contact with well elderly people, Health Visitors together with other members of the Primary Health Care Team have been involved in establishing well elderly screening programmes. Since the introduction of the G.P. contract in 1990 (DOH, 1990), which makes G.P.s responsible for ensuring regular and frequent assessment of elderly clients aged over 75 years, there has been a proliferation of well elderly screening programmes. The purpose of such programmes is to detect functional disabilities which may be impeding an elderly person's ability to remain independent and affecting their quality of life. It is not aimed at identifying specific medical conditions, but at uncovering the effects of disease and social circumstances (Robertson, 1991).

Finally, Health Visitors are involved in providing supportive care for elderly people. The aim of this work is to prevent further deterioration occurring in existing conditions and where possible, to aid rehabilitation. An example of this work is supporting carers of elderly dependants to ensure that they receive all the services and financial benefits available to help them in their caring role. This may involve regular respite care to enable carers to have a break from caring to recuperate their own physical and emotional health. Another example of supportive care is bereavement visiting where the Health Visitor assists individuals to work through the grief process to come to terms with their loss and to eventual grief resolution through supportive listening.

Case history

Mrs Cook is an elderly woman who lives alone. She came to the attention of the Health Visitor through the screening programme which had been established by the G.P. practice. In accordance with the G.P. contract, the practice are offering health screening to all clients aged over 75 years registered with the practice. In order to initiate contact with the well elderly population, the practice has been using the Edinburgh Birthday Card Scheme (Porter, 1987). Using this scheme a birthday card and letter are sent to all clients registered with the practice on their 75th, 80th and 85th birthdays together with a simple screening letter. Ideally, the practice should contact their well elderly population much earlier, such as from 65 years of age, but currently they do not have the resources to implement this. Earlier contact widens the scope for more preventive and health promotion work.

The screening letter inquires about such factors as help needed with housework and shopping, whether the person is unable to leave the house for whatever reason, problems previously not discussed with the doctor and access to help if needed. If the elderly person responds positively to more than one item or fails to return the letter then the Health Visitor visits them at home. The screening letter reduces unnecessary visits to elderly people who are not experiencing any problems and makes the screening of the well elderly population ·more manageable for the practice within their limited resources.

Mrs Cook had received the letter and birthday card on her 75th birthday. She was surprised to receive a card from her G.P. surgery but thought it was a nice gesture. She was last seen by the G.P. four years ago when she had shingles. The Health Visitor had contacted Mrs Cook to gain her permission to conduct a full health assessment and arrange a convenient time to call.

Mrs Cook has lived alone since the death of her husband ten years ago. She still lives in the family home which is a large three bedroomed detached house on the outskirts of a small village. She has three sons, but two have emigrated abroad and the third son lives far away. She has a close friend who calls weekly after collecting Mrs Cook's pension and bringing her shopping. Most of the neighbours are elderly people and are limited in the help they can offer.

Mrs Cook answers the door and the Health Visitor introduces herself and shows her identification card. Mrs Cook warmly welcomes her into the back room which is warm and cosy although the hall is quite chilly and dimly lit. Mrs Cook looks tired and drawn. The Health Visitor explains that on receiving her reply to the screening letter she would like to undertake a full health assessment to identify any problems which she may be able to help her with and to ensure that Mrs Cook is receiving all benefits and services to which she is entitled.

Mrs Cook is keen to participate in the assessment. Such an assessment involves inquiring about physical health status, social activities and relationships, lifestyle such as smoking, level of nutrition, mental health status, environmental factors such as housing, home safety, and a tactful enquiry into financial status.

The Health Visitor asks Mrs Cook about her hobbies and interests. She states that she enjoys reading and that a neighbour brings her books from the library once a month. However, she is finding small print books increasingly difficult to read. The Health Visitor asks when she last had her eyes tested. This had been over five years ago as she feels unable to manage the bus ride into town. She is informed of the need to have her eyes regularly tested at least every two years and that a domiciliary visiting service is provided by most opticians. In addition, large print books are available from the library and she may find these easier to read. Mrs Cook is concerned about the cost of glasses if these are needed. The Health Visitor tactfully discusses finances with Mrs Cook and it would seem that she may be eligible for income support. Mrs Cook is unsure whether she wants to claim, so the Health Visitor discusses all the additional benefits of receiving income support for example, free dental and optical care and leaves a leaflet with her. Many elderly people may be reluctant to accept what they see as charity and may need encouragement to claim that to which they are entitled. The Health Visitor will follow this up at the next visit and will help her apply for the benefit if she so wishes.

The Health Visitor then assesses Mrs Cook's physical health by asking her questions about all her bodily systems. Mrs Cook is in reasonably good health. She is not taking any prescribed medication although takes Ex-Lax every day to relieve constipation. The Health Visitor discusses ways of preventing constipation to try to avoid the need for daily medication. Long-term use of laxatives may render them ineffective.

Mrs Cook enjoys her food and enjoys cooking. The Health Visitor asks her to describe what she ate yesterday and whether this was a typical day's diet. Her diet is lacking in fibre in particular, very little fruit and vegetables and high in refined sugar such as cakes and biscuits. Mrs Cook reports that she dislikes fruit but could eat more vegetables and a bran-based cereal. As Mrs Cook is overweight the Health Visitor discusses her diet with her in detail, advising her to reduce her intake of cakes, biscuits and fatty foods and increase her intake of starchy foods such as bread and potatoes.

Mrs Cook then explains that for several months she has been limiting her fluid intake. This is because she has been finding it increasingly difficult to get to the toilet in time and has been moderately incontinent. She felt too embarrassed to talk to her G.P. about it and felt she could manage the situation herself. A considerable proportion of conditions in elderly people may be unknown to the G.P. As McClymont et al (1991) state the bulk of these conditions include urinary tract disorders, locomotor difficulties, foot problems, dementia and depression. The incontinence has become worse so that Mrs Cook has to go to the toilet almost hourly and has to get up three or four times during the night. She now does not feel confident to leave the house. The Health Visitor reassures her that incontinence is quite a common problem with elderly people and that help is available. Firstly, she explains to Mrs Cook that she will need to provide a specimen of urine for testing to eliminate a urinary tract infection. With her permission she will refer her to the District Continence Adviser at the Community Continence Clinic for a thorough assessment. After a thorough assessment Mrs Cook will be taught how to retrain her bladder so that she can hold on longer before going to the toilet. Whilst bladder training may take several months the outcome is usually good. In the meantime Mrs Cook is advised to drink at least six cups of fluid a day but to limit her fluid intake in the evenings. She is advised to increase her fibre intake to avoid constipation which may exacerbate her urinary incontinence and to try to lose some weight. She also discusses skin care and the importance of keeping the skin clean and dry.

In addition, the Health Visitor offers to provide Mrs Cook with a commode and incontinence pads. Mrs Cook is relieved that she has spoken to someone about her problem and willingly agrees for the referral to be made and accepts the offer of the commode and pads.

Mrs Cook talks much more openly now and seems more receptive to advice. She explains that she has hard skin and a painful corn on her foot and inquires about the possibility of chiropody treatment. The Health Visitor informs her that she is eligible for free chiropody although warns her that there is a long waiting list. Mrs Cook asks to be referred.

The Health Visitor then asks how Mrs Cook is managing in such a large house. She says 'the house really is too big for one person but it is so full of happy memories that I can't imagine living anywhere else'. She has closed off the two spare bedrooms and only heats the rooms she uses. The house is expensive to heat and the heating bills are a worry. The house is not centrally heated but heated by electric fires. The Health Visitor discusses with her the importance of adequate heating to prevent hypothermia and how she could receive help with insulating the house.

The Health Visitor remarks on the clothes drying in front of the electric fire. Mrs Cook is informed of the fire hazard and says that she has singed clothes in the past. This leads on to a discussion about home safety and whether she has a smoke alarm. She says that she does not and is informed of a scheme run by the local Age Concern office who will install a smoke alarm free of charge. She is given the contact name and says she will call. The Health Visitor continues to discuss home safety with Mrs Cook. This includes removing slip mats and trailing flexes and having adequate lighting in the hall. She says she has a non-slip mat in the bath and a bath rail. She has a safety chain on the door and a spyhole. She says that she does not open the door to strangers and is reminded to ask tradesmen and officials for their identity cards.

The house is quite isolated, being half a mile from the local shops in the village. Besides her close friend who calls regularly she has few visitors. She says she feels lonely at times and sometimes feels 'down'. The Health Visitor informs her of the local luncheon club and over 60s club for when the incontinence has improved and the possibility of arranging a voluntary visitor. Mrs Cook says that she would like to think about it.

The Health Visitor notices that Mrs Cook is getting tired. She summarises the main points of the visit and arranges to visit in three week's time. Visiting by appointment has been shown to be beneficial for elderly clients as it raises their morale and helps them cope with their problems if they know when the Health Visitor will next be calling (Luker, 1982). Following the visit the Health Visitor refers Mrs Cook to the chiropodist and to the District Continence Adviser.

The Health Visitor identifies her health needs as:

- inadequate intake of fibre and fluids
- urinary incontinence
- social isolation exacerbated by incontinence
- risk of falls
- being overweight
- limited income
- risk of hypothermia due to limited income
- failing eyesight
- corns and hard skin on her feet

Key aspects of health visiting with elderly people

1   identification of social isolation and mobilisation of services
2   prevention of accidents
3   prevention of hypothermia
4   nutritional advice
5   provision of information on benefits and services
6   health assessment

5 The Health Visitor and families with special needs

There are many families who experience interrelated social, economic and medical conditions which make them susceptible to illness and to disintegration as a unit. While most of health visiting is concerned with the functioning family, there is an increasing number of families which are faced with a multiplicity of problems such as violence, unemployment and disability. These problems are long-term and often require intensive health and social services support.

As a student in the community you are seeing a range of families of many different types and with many different problems and needs. One aspect of family life which you may meet is that of violence. Violence within a family context is not a new or unknown phenomenon, and it occurs across all social classes and cultures.

Essentially violence can be seen as a misuse of physical and economic power and therefore the main victims within a family context are women, children and the elderly.

Why do we find violence within families?

1 The amount of time spent within the family makes it more likely that violence can occur between members.
2 The activities and interests of the family provide opportunity for conflict; added to this is the overlap or competition of these activities, e.g. what TV programme to watch – or how money should be allocated.
3 Family members have a high level of emotional involvement which can create tensions.
4 There is a presumed right of family members to influence each other and exert control over actions and behaviour.
5 Members represent differing outlooks of age and sex and roles are assigned on these criteria, not on interest or competency.
6 We have a lack of choice in whether we belong to a family. There is limited availability of escape despite divorce.
7 The private nature of families excludes outside contact and makes it easier for violence to take place without censure.

Child abuse

One type of violence within the family is that of child abuse, which falls into four categories, though these often overlap:

Physical injury: Typically, the abused child is a toddler or baby, although older children can be at risk. The child may have bruising, or tissue damage; burns and scalds are often seen and there may be evidence of fractures. Some injuries are life-threatening.

Neglect: may also be manifest with the baby failing to thrive because of inadequate diet. The child may be insufficiently clothed and the home may be dirty and cold.

Emotional abuse: may occur even if there is good physical care. The child may be terrorised and rejected, and made to feel worthless.

Sexual abuse: Incest, sexual molestation and rape within families are still taboo subjects for many people. In families where these problems occur, they are often hidden and the guilty party (usually the male) is protected.

What factors lead to child abuse?

Child abuse does not result from one single cause, and it is necessary to examine a number of predisposing factors.

Parents who abuse their children often suffered abuse or emotional deprivation themselves as children. People from such backgrounds may marry people with similar experiences or may marry to escape from a bad home situation (Carver, 1978), and because they are often emotionally as well as physically immature, they are not able to cope with the difficulties of parenthood.

Although abusing parents may come from any socio-economic group they tend to have certain characteristics. They are often isolated emotionally and physically, with little support from relatives or the social services. Many have interrelated problems such as unemployment affecting their marriage, housing, economic stability and relationships.

Medical problems leading to child abuse may centre on the parent or child. Some parents who are ill or even have minor complaints such as anaemia are less able to cope with child-rearing. There may be a history of marital or sexual difficulties which intensify their frustrations. Parents who are treated with tranquillisers or antidepressants are also at risk of abusing children, as these drugs remove inhibition.

The abused child is more likely to have been the product of an unwanted pregnancy or premature or difficult delivery. There is often a history of childhood illness or handicap with long periods of separation affecting the parent-child bonding. The child may have feeding difficulties, be very unsettled with long periods of crying and present as a 'difficult baby' who is 'hard to rear'.

Parental expectations Abusing parents may have unreal expectations of their children. These parents have little understanding of child development and punish the child for failing to live up to their impossible demands.

Social factors While not all abusing parents suffer from social stress there is no doubt that for many parents the burdens of poverty, unemployment and deprived environments can put them more at risk of abusing their children.

Case history

The Health Visitor has been visiting Joan Kerr for 18 months since the birth of her daughter, Cathy. Joan is 18 years old and has been in the care of the local authority for most of her life. She is currently living with Terry, aged 20, an unemployed lorry driver, but this is not a stable relationship. Joan has cohabited with a series of men over the past two years. Cathy's father is unknown.

Joan and Terry live in a poorly furnished council flat which is damp, noisy and difficult to heat. The couple have large bills for gas and electricity which are almost impossible for them to meet out of their social security benefits. Although Joan is very proud of Cathy and tries hard to make ends meet she is very dispirited and sees little way out of her situation. Terry has a history of petty crime and is frequently aggressive when the social worker calls; although he seems to accept the Health Visitor, he is very uncommunicative. Joan appears quite afraid of him but has never indicated that he has been violent to her or Cathy.

The Health Visitor is in frequent contact with the social worker about them as they are in danger of having their heating cut off. The social worker and Health Visitor recognise that there is a possibility of violence within the family and are trying to prevent this by frequent visiting and offering help to relieve the stress of poverty and poor housing, e.g. obtaining grants from voluntary organisations or referring to the Welfare Rights Office for comprehensive advice on social security benefits.

Cathy has not been immunised and is never brought to the baby clinic. Developmental assessments carried out at home by the Health Visitor indicate that she appears small for her age and lacking in stimulation. She has frequent colds and infections. The nutritional state of the family is poor as there is little money for food and Joan and Terry do not cook, relying on convenience food such as bread and chips.

One day when the Health Visitor calls she finds Cathy with bruising on her cheeks and a bruised lip. At first Joan replies that Cathy fell, but then after some time says that Terry hit Cathy because she was unable to use the potty and had soiled her nappy (an occurrence quite normal at this age). Terry has left the house and his whereabouts are unknown. The Health Visitor decides that this is a definite case of child abuse and her main aim must be to protect the child from further harm. She has no legal powers to take the child into care; that is the function of the social worker. These are actions that she can take:

1   Contact the Senior Nurse, G.P. and social worker to arrange a case conference as soon as possible to discuss the future of the family.
2   Write a full report describing the state of the child and social background.
3   Ask the G.P. to call to make sure there is no other injury or ask the mother to bring the child to the Health Centre or Accident and Emergency Department.
4   Continue to visit in conjunction with the social worker to prevent any further abuse.

Various factors had alerted the health and social services to the possible danger of child abuse in this family:

• Joan had been abused as a child and has been in care.
• Lack of extended family or support.
• Unstable, potentially aggressive relationship.
• Cohabiting male who is not the child's father.
• Unrealistic expectations of the child by Terry concerning toilet training.
• Severe social stress.

How might the Health Visitor help prevent child abuse?

1   Educating young people about the frustrations and difficulties of parenting.
2   Antenatal preparation for the emotional aspects of childbirth and childrearing.
3   Identifying potentially abusing parents and helping towards relieving stress.
4   Providing support and help for abusive and potentially abusive parents in conjunction with other agencies such as NSPCC.

5   Maintaining an effective record keeping and referral system for herself and to link with other agencies such as social workers.

Incidence of child abuse: It is very difficult to give accurate figures but Kempe and Kempe (1978) suggest that 6 infants per 1,000 are battered. There are over 100 known deaths per year from abuse. The incidence of incest and child sexual abuse is unknown but it has been estimated that 1 in 4 women have been sexually molested in childhood, usually by male family members (Wilson, 1983).

Violence against women

Health Visitors are visiting families in which women are the victims of violence. How might Health Visitors recognise abuse?

Abuse should be suspected when a woman presents with multiple injuries, when she is injured while pregnant or has a history of multiple or self-induced abortions; when she presents with persistent or vague medical complaints, when she has attempted suicide or persistently uses tranquillisers and shows anxiety and depression.

Women who have been abused by violence make multiple visits to the medical and psychiatric services for general health problems which superficially appear to be unrelated to abuse, but which are as much a part of the battering syndrome as the physical injury (Orr, 1984).

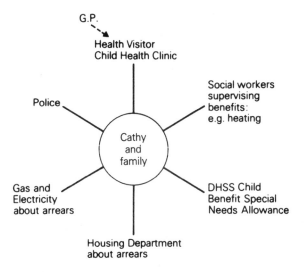

Fig. 5.1 Agencies in contact with Cathy's family

Many of these factors can be seen in the following history of Mrs Lane and fit into the second stage of the Battering Syndrome.

Three stages of the Battering Syndrome:

1st stage: Suffers repeated physical injuries.
2nd stage: Presents with more serious psychosocial problems along with their physical injuries. They are often referred to the psychiatric services at this stage.
3rd stage: Presents with severe medical or mental health problems and may have turned to self-abuse or suicide attempts.

Case history

The Health Visitor had been visiting Mrs Lane since the birth of her daughter, Elizabeth, four years ago, but on all visits she had appeared distant and had never been particularly welcoming. In that time Mrs Lane had had two miscarriages. The Lanes' lived in a large detached house, which was well furnished and always immaculately clean and tidy. Mr Lane, aged 45, was a bank manager and Mrs Lane, aged 32, had been his secretary until their marriage. Their G.P. had expressed concern to the Health Visitor about the increasing frequency with which Mrs Lane was attending the surgery presenting with a range of physical and emotional complaints such as headaches, pains and feelings of anxiety. The G.P. and the Health Visitor both felt that Mrs Lane had a major problem which she was reluctant to discuss and it was agreed that the Health Visitor would call as soon as possible. The Health Visitor was planning a visit in any case because Elizabeth was now four and due to be seen before starting school to check on developmental progress and immunisation.

It took Mrs Lane a long time to open the door. When she did it was clear that she was agitated, had been crying and appeared to have some difficulty moving her upper body. She was reluctant to let the Health Visitor in and stood in the hall for a few minutes until the Health Visitor said, 'Would you like to talk about it, I might be able to help.' At that Mrs Lane started to cry, raised her jumper to show a large bruise and lacerations on her left side and said, 'He beats me but he'll kill me if I tell anyone, I don't know what to do, there's nowhere I can go, I'm so ashamed.'

The Health Visitor sat next to Mrs Lane and listened for a long time as she talked of her life. Her husband had started abusing her one year after their marriage and when she was pregnant he had kicked her and given her a black eye. He seemed to resent her pregnancy and Mrs Lane blamed his assaults on her for the two miscarriages. Over the last year the beatings had become more frequent and she did not know what to do.

What help can the Health Visitor offer Mrs Lane? She can offer information about the availability of local women's refuges which are set up by Women's Aid Groups to provide shelter for the battered woman and her children. She can also inform Mrs Lane of her legal rights and suggest she contact a solicitor. If Mrs Lane does not feel able or is afraid to take any action then the Health Visitor must respect that decision and offer support and counselling to Mrs Lane. In many cases women choose to stay for the sake of their children. Some women will understandably be reluctant to take action because of the difficulties involved in leaving violent men and of finding alternative accommodation and income. Abusing men will often continue to harass and make life untenable for the victim by destroying any new accommodation and threatening violence to a helping family or friend.

What is the extent of violence against women? As in the case of child abuse it is difficult to be sure of the size of the problem; however, there is enough evidence to suggest that it is considerable. A study of women's refuges in England and Wales gives us some idea of the numbers of women seeking help (Binney *et al.*, 1981). Taking into account 150 refuges in England and Wales, 11 400 women and 20 850 children sought help between 1977 and 1978.

The figures in Table 5.1 show that many women seeking help had been battered for a long period of time. Their ages ranged from under 20 years to 71 years of age.

Table 5.1 Length of time before battered women seek help

Length of time battered	Number of women	Percentage of women
Less than 3 years	172	27
3 to under 6 years	165	26
6 to under 10 years	140	22
10 years or more	159	25
TOTAL	636	100

Families experiencing unemployment

'In the eighties unemployed girls who've never experienced economic independence are doing the only thing they can – having babies, either getting married or not, but often staying with their Mum and Dad and quite soon getting a council house. They never consider an abortion,

often don't use contraception. They want children. Of course they do.
There just isn't anything else.'

Beatrix Campbell (1984)
Wigan Pier Revisited

What Beatrix Campbell describes about the effects of poverty
and unemployment in Wigan can be found in many other towns
throughout the United Kingdom. Unemployment affects people in
many ways, causing loss of status and feelings of worthlessness. The
reality of long-term unemployment can destroy or distort family
relationships leading to an increase in the incidence of alcoholism,
ill health and family violence.

One of the features of unemployment in the 1990s is that it affects
a wide range of people. Traditionally unemployment has been a
feature of the lives of unskilled or semi-skilled workers but now
skilled and professional people are also experiencing unemployment.
In addition Sinfield (1981) describes how those in work are affected
by high unemployment because of insecurity of work, fear of redundancy and cutbacks in overtime.

Women who have traditionally been employed in low paid and
part-time work are very vulnerable to changes in employment
patterns. In addition the social and health services which are cut
back not only affect them as workers but also as consumers. If we
take the case of the cut back in home care assistants, for example,
we can see that women are losing the jobs of home care assistants and
in many cases having to increase their private contribution to caring
for aged or infirmed relatives. Health Visitors working in areas of
high unemployment therefore need to be aware of the stress within
families and of her role in helping them to obtain all the benefits they
are due. The Health Visitor also has to be aware that, as in the case
of young girls described by Campbell, it is simply not enough to offer
contraceptive advice. People will make decisions about health issues
which are closely related to the wider social and economic issues and
therefore changes are needed in society to improve health e.g. to
reduce poverty and improve levels of nutrition.

Case history

Judy Rogers has a three month baby girl called Tracey. Judy is 17
years old and lives with her parents and three older brothers in a
small terrace house. The baby's father is abroad and does not know
of Tracey's birth. Judy left school when she became pregnant. She
has applied for six jobs but there is little hope of obtaining employment in her local area. Judy's parents have been very supportive
although initially they were distressed when Judy told them she was
pregnant.

While they love the baby there have been great difficulties with overcrowding and Judy has been given a council flat in a very deprived estate in another part of the town.

The Health Visitor considers Judy a high priority and would visit her frequently. She puts Judy in contact with voluntary bodies such as Gingerbread (a group for one parent families) and would try to get the baby into day care if Judy got a job.

The Health Visitor considers Judy at risk because she is a young inexperienced mother isolated geographically from her family. Despite help from her parents, Judy is finding it very difficult to furnish her flat and the Health Visitor has contacted the Voluntary Services Agency for help with essential furnishings.

Judy seems to have unrealistic expectations of how she will manage on a low income and is given help with budgeting. At first Judy was relieved to have her own home and be away from her parents but increasingly she is feeling the strain of caring for a young baby on her own. There are few neighbours with whom Judy wants to make friends and the area is not safe at night to be out alone. The Health Visitor invites her to a mother and baby group at the clinic and introduces her to some other young mothers on the estate. Judy's problem may mean her returning to her parents but that will not be satisfactory in the long term.

Services and benefits for one parent families: Income Support, one parent benefit, Child benefit, milk tokens and vitamins, help with maternity needs such as baby clothes.

The family with a handicapped child

When you are visiting you may meet a range of people with handicapping conditions. By handicap we mean any factor, physical, social or emotional, which prevents the child reaching their full potential. Sometimes the term 'special need' is used instead of 'handicap'. Listen to what is used when you are with the Community Nurse.

Out of 20 children, one will have some abnormality or defect. Some of these abnormalities are obvious at birth. They may be minor ones, such as extra fingers or toes or birth marks, or they may be much more serious, such as spina bifida, club feet, cleft palate and hare lip, or Down's syndrome.

Most handicaps however are not obvious at birth. All babies are examined by the doctor, midwife and Health Visitor during the first two weeks, and a special blood test is performed to find out whether or not the babies suffer from two rare diseases called phenylketonuria and hypothyroidism. The majority of handicaps only become obvious as the baby grows, and for this reason it is important to ensure that the baby is examined regularly. These examinations may be carried out in a hospital department, in a G.P.'s surgery, or in a local authority child health clinic by the Health Visitor.

One of the functions of the Health Visitor is to identify children who are not reaching their developmental milestones. All children of course do not develop according to text books! Many will be walking sooner than others for example and the developmental schedules are used only as a guideline. Many normal babies who are late at milestones may have been premature or ill or may have difficult or disturbed backgrounds.

But children with real handicaps, visual or hearing defects, cerebral palsy or mental retardation, are also slow in their development, and it is most important that they should be diagnosed and have appropriate treatment at the earliest possible age. Parents know their children better than anyone else. It is the parents that notice and fear that their baby may be deaf, mentally retarded or may squint, and the Health Visitor must take very seriously what the parents tell her about their child. Parents can be encouraged to help their children and are often very anxious to know what to do.

The slow developer can be helped by appropriate activity, by stimulating play, and by being talked to. For the handicapped child there are special facilities, such as special nursery groups or a trained teacher who may visit the home. Voluntary societies and local authorities may provide trained visitors for children who are deaf, blind or who suffer from cerebral palsy. But these visitors rely on the parents to carry out exercises and training in the home, and the full burden falls on them. The Health Visitor, therefore, has a major role in supporting the parents as well as advising them on issues such as discipline.

For the more serious handicaps, there are special societies that parents can join, where they meet other parents of children with similar handicaps who may employ specially trained social workers and who may run special nurseries and schools for severely handicapped children. But the majority of handicapped children do not come into this category. Their handicaps are slight, and with appropriate treatment can be overcome. For these children the local health authority makes full provision. Parent counselling is provided at the clinic and in the home. Special training may be provided in nurseries, and where necessary, special education may be available from the age of two.

Key roles of Health Visitor

- provide information for parents on the best way of helping the child
- liaise with hospital, schools and social workers
- put parents in contact with voluntary agencies

- ensure that all social security benefits are being claimed
- enable parents to talk openly about their feelings
- advise on childhood management
- recognise the stress and help parents and other family members to cope with the situation
- provide the opportunity for parents to meet others in similar situations
- provide all appropriate aids for the child
- ensure that respite care is offered to the parents

Test yourself

1 What handicapped children does your Health Visitor have in her caseload?
2 Are there any voluntary societies for handicapped children in your area?
3 Are there any self-help groups?
4 Is there provision for battered women in the area?
5 How many children does your Health Visitor have on the at risk register for child abuse?
6 What is the level of unemployment in the area?
7 How many one parent families does the Health Visitor have in her caseload?

6 The role of the District Nurse in the care of elderly people

'Instead of retiring from life, I am pleased and excited to be able to recycle and redirect my goals. I continue to realise that old age is a time of great fulfillment – personal fulfillment when all the loose ends of life can be gathered together.'

Maggie Kuhn, 80 years old,
Leader of the Gray Panthers,
in Bauman *et al.*, 1981

We are currently experiencing a change in the age structure of our population never before seen in human history. An emotive phrase – the greying of the nation – is used to describe it. The change is of course the ever increasing numbers of elderly people, more especially of the older elderly. In 1991 there were 8.75 million people over the age of 65 years in Britain, the government statistics definition of elderly. Fig. 6.1 shows the known and predicted rise in the elderly population between 1921 and 2021.

The rise in the numbers of elderly is caused by the continued

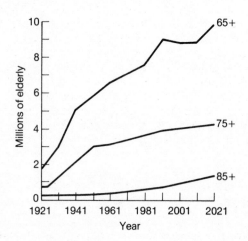

Fig. 6.1 Elderly population in Britain

improvement in the life expectancy of people in Britain (see Table 6.1).

Table 6.1 Expectation of life: Further number of years which a person may expect to live. (*Source*: OPCS, 1992)

		1901	1931	1961	1981	1991	2001
Males	Age						
	0	45.5	58.4	67.9	70.8	73.2	74.5
	1	53.6	62.1	68.9	70.5	72.8	74.0
	10	50.4	55.6	60.0	62.0	64.0	65.2
	20	41.7	46.7	50.4	52.3	54.2	55.4
	40	26.1	29.5	31.5	33.2	35.1	36.2
	60	13.3	14.4	15.0	16.3	17.6	18.7
	80	4.9	4.9	5.2	5.7	6.3	7.0
Females							
	0	49.0	62.4	73.8	76.8	78.8	79.9
	1	55.8	65.1	74.2	76.6	78.3	79.3
	10	52.7	58.6	65.6	67.8	69.5	70.5
	20	44.1	49.6	55.7	57.9	59.6	60.6
	40	28.3	32.4	36.5	38.5	40.0	41.0
	60	14.6	16.4	19.0	20.8	21.9	22.7
	80	5.3	5.4	6.3	7.5	8.3	8.8

One has only to think of many of the world's political figures to appreciate that many people over 65 are still mentally and physically active. It is usual, therefore, to consider the elderly as two groups, the young elderly, 65–75 years, and the old elderly, 75 plus. It is certainly the case that this second group (75+) does experience a high incidence of ill health and reduced mobility as compared to younger people. The increased expenditure for personal social services (Fig. 6.2), clearly demonstrates this point. Indeed over the age of 85 the majority (66%) of people are to some extent ill or disabled and 10% of them are in need of a considerable amount of nursing care. Only 5% of these older people are in hospital at any one time. The overwhelming proportion of the nursing this group needs is therefore provided within the community. Fig. 6.3 shows the incidence of chronic illness recorded in 1991.

Who provides nursing care for the elderly in the community?

One of the first things you will notice when going out with the District Nurse is that most of her patients are old people. Approximately one

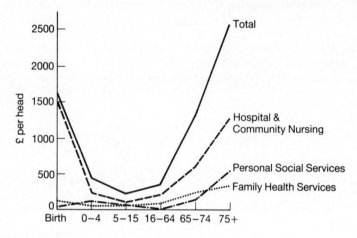

Fig. 6.2 Expenditure on Health and Personal Social Services. (*Source*: OPCS, 1992.)

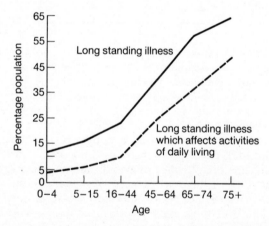

Fig. 6.3 Chronic illness reported in 1991 General Household Survey. (*Source*: OPCS Monitor (1992). General Household Survey Preliminary Reports for 1991.)

million old people are visited by District Nurses per year. These visits account for three-quarters of the District Nurse's total patient contact time and almost half (44%) of their work is with people over 75 years old.

Yet despite the fact that the District Nurse spends most of her time with elderly patients, the community nursing service is meeting only a small percentage of this group's needs (Table 6.2). It is estimated that only 6.2% of elderly people are in contact with a District Nurse (the figure rises to 20% of those over 85 years old). This still leaves the overwhelming majority of elderly people without District Nursing assistance despite the fact that we know that many of them are ill or disabled.

Table 6.2 Contact with elderly people. (*Source*: General Household Survey, 1981)

	percentage
Visit G.P.'s surgery	24
G.P. visited at home	10
Seen District Nurse or Health Visitor	6
Chiropodist	10
Home help	9
Meals on Wheels	3
Day Centre	5

Families do care

Contrary to widely held myths, therefore, families do care for their elderly relatives – indeed they bear the major burden of this care in the community. It is important to remember, however, that as a result of the changes in family structure, e.g. fewer children, the increasing numbers of people reaching old age and the fact that many children have to move away from home for work, the 'carer' is likely to be an equally old spouse. Fig. 6.4 breaks down the types of household in which elderly people live into five categories and shows this to be the case for 39% of elderly people in 1986. As Cresswell and Pasker (1972) noted,

> 'Those who look after the dependant are small in numbers and old in years. They may well need a lot of looking after themselves if the whole concept of community care is not going to crumble. The frail are propping up the frailer.'

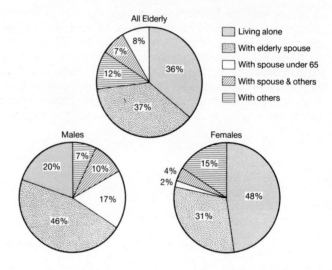

Fig. 6.4   Type of household in which elderly people live. (*Source*: OPCS, 1989.)

Case history

One example of this is given by Mrs Smith who has looked after her husband single-handedly ever since his stroke five years ago.

'Mr Smith is 81 and I am 80. We live alone and we've always been independent – the neighbours never ask "Do you want an errand doing?" so I never ask – I do it myself. I do things I never thought I'd have to do. I even have to wipe his bottom when he is on the commode. Sometimes I think I can't go on, but I know there are lots of people in the same position – it's a terrible strain, with the diabetes. In a sense I have to neglect myself to look after him. I have to do everything. I can hardly keep my eyes open, I'm dead weary. He's no help to himself at all. I was up every hour last night. I am surprised myself how I've kept up. It's not as though I'm young is it?'

Many older people, like Mrs Smith, believe very firmly in trying to manage on their own. They often accept a considerable amount of ill health or disability as an inevitable aspect of ageing. Consequently by the time the District Nurse or other members of the Primary Health Care Team become involved, both the carer and the patient are often exhausted and at the end of their tether.

As can be seen from Fig. 6.5 a) and b) there is a belief that there is a large amount of unreported disability amongst old people at home.

This belief in high levels of unreported disease amongst the elderly may be exaggerated (Bowling, 1989). It would seem that where a major disease is present it is usually known to the G.P., but many of the disabling conditions that restrict a person's ability to remain independent and thereby put a great burden on the carer are social and nursing problems.

In recognition of the problem of unreported need among the elderly, Primary Health Care Teams are required under the 1990

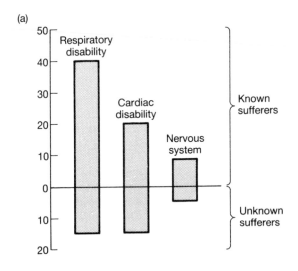

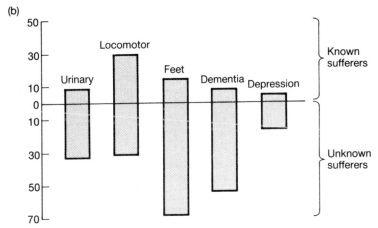

Fig. 6.5 a) and b) Unreported disability among old people at home. (*Source*: Williamson, J., 1981.)

G.P. contract to carry out routine screening programmes for this patient group.

The ageing process is associated with increased frailty and vulnerability to ill health but many other factors contribute to the high incidence of disability and handicap experienced by the elderly. The District Nurse's role is to identify and relieve these contributing factors where possible, as patients and relatives may dismiss relievable conditions as just old age:

Disease may be due to or accentuated by the lack of appropriate 'aids', e.g. glasses for the visually impaired, hearing aids for the deaf, appropriate footwear and good chiropody which may significantly increase mobility, etc.

Social factors. For example isolation may lead to depression and poor housing and poverty (often linked to age) to malnutrition and/or hypothermia.

Disease, disability and social problems of the elderly are all interrelated (Fig. 6.6); e.g. a mild stroke that leaves the patient incontinent of urine will, if not relieved or properly managed, increase the patient's isolation – no one wants an incontinent person in a bin go club and equally, the patient is too embarrassed to go out anyway. If the old person is living in poor accommodation with numerous stairs and loose carpets and has arthritis, the combination of the disease and the inappropriate environment will accentuate the patient's immobility and hence ability to maintain his independence.

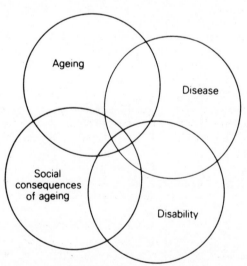

Fig. 6.6 The four processes of old age. (Adapted from Wilcock, G. *et al.*, 1982)

Assessment of the elderly

We have noted that:

1   the elderly, especially those over 75 years old, are likely to be suffering some degree of ill health
2   their supporters/carers are likely to be equally old and frail
3   because of old people's health beliefs and attitudes, they are likely not to have reported all their health problems to their G.P.

Consequently the District Nurse's assessment of an elderly person has to be particularly thorough. The District Nurse's even more than usual must assess the carer's health and the available support network as well as the patient. In addition to the basic routine physical, psychological and social assessments of both patient and carer as individuals, it is useful to estimate the coping ability of the family as a single unit. If, for example, the patient is receiving excellent care but the carer is very resentful about the situation, the family unit is not coping fully and is therefore 'at risk'.

Freeman and Heinrich (1981) outline one approach, i.e. the Family Coping Index, on which to base this assessment.

1   *Physical independence.* How far can the family unit manage the activities of daily living? The patient may be immobile, but if the carer is able to move him e.g. in a wheelchair then the family unit is reasonably physically independent.
2   *Therapeutic competence.* How far can the family unit carry out the procedures or treatments prescribed e.g. giving medicine correctly, using aids and appliances such as walking frames, carrying out exercises and/or preparing an appropriate diet.
3   *Knowledge of health condition.* Does the family unit recognise disease and disability as separate from the ageing process? What is their level of knowledge about the particular problems of ill health they are experiencing and any tests or hospital admissions planned for the future?
4   *Application of principles of personal and general hygiene and safety.* How far does the family unit understand and carry out these principles, e.g. disposal of dirty dressings, or need to heat house adequately.
5   *How does the family as a unit feel about their health care and the services they are receiving?* To what extent are they prepared to take preventive measures to maintain their well being? Would they like more or fewer services e.g. home helps, laundry service, more information about the disease, etc. Remember that an elderly person's attitudes are based on past experiences and attitudes of a

different period.

6　*Emotional competence.* How far is the family unit able to cope with the stress of illness and disability? How realistic are they about the future? Is there anger/resentment about having to cope with the patient? Is any member mentally frail, handicapped or ill?

7　*Family living patterns.* How do the family members get on together? Does one person make all the decisions? Was the patient the dominant family member prior to their illness? How has this affected the family relationships?

8　*Physical environment.* Has the house adequate facilities, heating, etc.? What is the immediate neighbourhood like – where are the nearest shops, post office, etc.? What public transport is available? Are the streets safe? Is there a significant amount of theft or attacks on old people in the area?

9　*Use of community resources.* Is the family unit aware of and in receipt of all the services and benefits for which they are eligible (e.g. constant attendance allowance, mobility allowance, rate rebates, etc.)? Do they use the local facilities e.g. luncheon clubs, bingo halls? Do they belong to local groups, e.g. church, pensioners clubs, library, good neighbour schemes? Do they know how to get help promptly, e.g. Doctor/District Nurse's telephone number, police or social workers?

Although the above assessment considers the needs of a family unit, we have seen that many old people live alone and in that context the 'family unit' is more accurately described as a 'care unit' which may consist of the old person and their neighbour or home help.

The prime focus of the District Nurse's work with the elderly is health education – maintaining self-esteem. Clearly whatever the primary diagnosis with which an old person is labelled, e.g. arthritis or leg ulcer, this will not be the only challenge to their state of well-being. We have noted that old age is marked by multiple pathology and sensory losses and the additional complicating symptoms of physical frailty and reduced mobility. Psychological stamina is also reduced and the elderly therefore adapt to change and stress with difficulty. The death of friends and relatives, the fear of injury or attack, an inappropriate environment and the negative view of ageing found in our youth-orientated society all contribute to a decline in their self-esteem. When illness is added to these stresses, with its resulting increased dependence on others, the problem is magnified. Low self-esteem and the inability to do things for themselves leads, for many, to a sense of helplessness, hopelessness, depression and death (Fig. 6.7).

District Nurses are well aware that however competent they may be in caring for the physical needs of their patients, unless they are able to maintain the old person's self-esteem, their work is in vain.

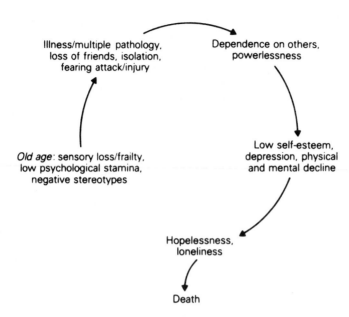

Fig. 6.7 The vicious circle of ageing. (Adapted from Fitzgerald Miller, J., 1983)

Health education of the elderly can be identified therefore as any action that maximises the patient's control over his life and thus improves his sense of well-being. It may be teaching about diet, medication or exercise or how to apply for benefits, etc. or just allowing the elderly people to express their fears and talk about their life. The District Nurse also always knows that although she is a welcome support to the old people, she must never treat them as children.

Health education and the elderly – the District Nurse's role:

Primary Prevention: preventive education, particularly directed to the elderly carers of the patient e.g. need for rest and relaxation, avoidance of back strain, home safety, wise use of available resources/services.
Secondary Prevention: screening for unreported needs to treat before a crisis occurs. Bereavement visiting is an important part of the District Nurse's role in secondary prevention.
Tertiary Prevention: when illness or disability has occurred and maintenance and rehabilitation is the aim i.e. restoring patients to their fullest physical, mental and social capabilities within the limits of their disability.

With the Government committed to maintaining the elderly, both sick and well, in their own homes, the District Nurse is – and will be even more so in the future – at the sharp end of a policy that depends more than anything else on helping people to look after their own health and/or maximise their comfort and independence. It is the health education aspect of the District Nurse's work with the elderly that is most likely to achieve this goal.

Some problems commonly faced by the elderly

Problems associated with diet

Malnutrition. Although malnutrition is not common in the United Kingdom a survey of people over 70 years old found that 12% of the men and 8% of the women were malnourished (DHSS, 1980). The survey also indicated certain medical and social conditions that are associated with malnutrition in old people. When she identifies cases of malnutrition, the District Nurse will involve the other members of the Primary Health Care Team to assess and alleviate the underlying problem (Fig. 6.8).

Medical and social conditions associated with malnutrition.   Partial gastrectomy, chronic bronchitis and emphysema, confusion, Depression, dental problems (failure to use dentures), difficulty in swallowing, housebound, no regular cooked meals, Social class IV & V, receiving Supplementary Benefit (*Source*: DHSS, 1980).

Obesity. Often, old people, especially those living alone or with an elderly carer, subsist largely on tea and toast or other foods high in carbohydrate. Consequently many, particularly women, are obese despite being malnourished in relation to their vitamins, mineral and protein requirements. One can postulate a number of reasons for this, for example simple preference for sweet starchy foods, lack of money to buy fruits and meat, lack of incentive to cook 'proper' meals, etc.

Unfortunately – given that eating is one of the pleasures of life freely available to the elderly – an old person with reduced mobility requires fewer calories than more active younger people.

Obesity in the elderly is a serious problem. It increases the person's immobility making them more vulnerable to chest infections, heart disease, pressure sores, diabetes, etc. The problems of bad feet, arthritis and poor wound healing are also increased by obesity.

The District Nurse will advise old people on dieting, reducing fats, sugars and carbohydrate, and if appropriate advise on ways of taking more exercise. It is important not to encourage too fast a weight loss as this could have adverse effects such as hypotension, exhaustion and confusion. Slow and steady is the aim.

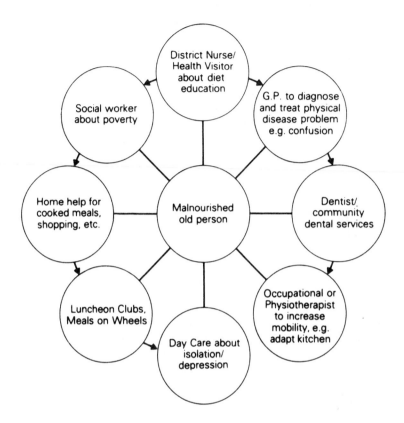

Fig. 6.8 The role of the Primary Health Care Team in malnutrition

Constipation. Many old people are extremely concerned with their bowels. Although it should be explained that frequent regular bowel movements are not 'normal' – especially if one is eating very little – the need to avoid constipation must also be stressed. Depression, drugs, dehydration and disease (e.g. cancer of the rectum) can all cause constipation. Elderly people tend to eat a diet low in fibre and take very little exercise, both of which are contributing factors. Constipation is not only unpleasant for the individual but aggravates any tendency to haemorrhoids. Faecal impaction (extreme constipation) leads to faecal overflow that may be confused with diarrhoea by the patient and treated with constipating medicine, making matters worse. Apart from re-educating the family on diet, etc., the constipation must be treated with laxatives, enemas or manual removal. It is important to remember that old people should always be attended at this time as the patient frequently feels weak and dizzy and may fall as he attempts to reach the commode or lavatory.

Problems of medication

As a result of ageing (e.g. lower metabolic rate, reduced blood flow to kidneys, liver and brain), old people tolerate drugs less easily than the young. The elderly are also, because of their multiple pathology, on a large number of medicines and may in addition be taking pills that are bought over the counter or pills that should have been discontinued. Non-compliance, i.e. not taking what has been prescribed when it should be taken, is a common problem among this patient group. Studies of elderly people in the community have found that less than half take their medicines exactly as prescribed and make a large number of potentially serious errors (Wade & Bowling, 1986).

Old people's medications, their reactions to it and their understanding of when and how to take their pills must be carefully monitored by the District Nurse. One District Nurse found an old lady's suppositories by the back door and was told by the patient that 'the doctor said I should put them in the back passage and leave them there!' Careful and repeated explanations with the use of memory joggers are clearly important aids of avoiding inappropriate medication. The use of child proof containers should be avoided – they are usually 'old person proof' as well! In cases where the old person is taking a number of drugs at various times the District Nurse will inform the G.P. who may be able to reassess the patient and adjust the medication.

Hypothermia

Drugs (e.g. sedatives or alcohol) may potentiate hypothermia (the condition in which the central body temperature drops below 35°C) in an old person. Certain disease states such as myxoedema also increase the risk of hypothermia. In old people however it is more commonly the result of:

1   reduced sensitivity to cold (i.e. the person does not feel cold).
2   The ageing body is less able to adjust to changes in temperature (i.e. impaired temperature regulating mechanism).
3   the old person may in fact feel the cold but resist putting on the heating because of the cost involved.

Where an old person is at risk of hypothermia the District Nurse works closely with the members of the Primary Health Care Team to find a solution (Fig 6.9).

Points to consider when caring for an old person:

1 Be aware of your own negative stereotypes of ageing and avoid treating the old as 'simple' or 'childlike' for example, use the full name initially not first name.
2 Adapt to the old persons' communication needs, talk face-to-face clearly, not shouting, allow time for them to answer, repeat explanations, etc.
3 Emphasise the positive to maintain self-esteem – not what they can't do but what they can do!
4 Use 'aid memoires' e.g. exercise or positioning charts, pill-taking charts or special dispensers, role play.
5 Obtain appropriate benefits, aids and equipment to maximise

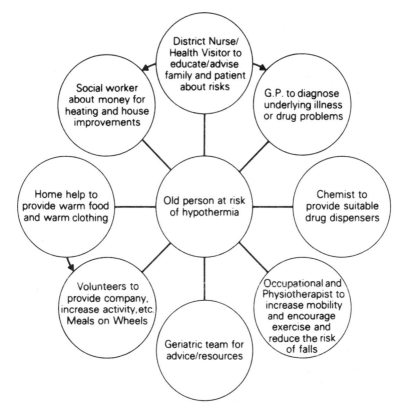

Fig. 6.9 The role of the Primary Health Care Team in hypothermia

mobility and independence.

6   Watch out for hazards, unsafe or cold homes.

7   Utilise the resources of the Primary Health Care Teams, the Specialist Geriatric Teams and Community Resources.

8   Support the carers and praise their efforts.

The elderly are the same individuals they were when they were young – indeed if you ask them how old they feel inside many are still in the prime of their youth. The role of the District Nurse is to enable them to express their sense of youth and individuality as fully as possible.

Test yourself

1   What percentage of the population in your area is over 65 years old? Is this number expected to increase or decrease in the future?

2   What facilities are there for older people in your area?

3   Who cares for the dependent elderly people in your area?

4   What is the prime focus of the District Nurse's work with older people?

5   How do you feel about growing old? What are the things you look forward to, what are the things you fear?

7 The role of the District Nurse in the care of the dying person and their family

'I don't want to die,' our daughter Jane said, when she learned at the age of 25 that she had cancer. But in the months which followed she proved that dying need not be the dreaded experience most of us imagine. Far from being the defeat it is usually thought to be, her death was a kind of victory – a battle won against pain and terror.

Zorza, R. & V. (1980)

Jane Zorza died of cancer at an age when most people justifiably anticipate at least a half a century more of active life (only 3.6% of deaths occur between the ages of 15 and 44 years old). Today nearly three-quarters of our population die when they are past 65 years of age – many of them well past. The fact remains, however, that although most of us will die in our old age, we must all die eventually. Life, as it is said, is a terminal condition. For most people death is something frightening, especially if associated with cancer, not to be talked about, not even to be thought about. As community nurses we are privileged to be with, learn from and help dying people and their families. It is not an easy task but it is possibly the most important one in nursing. You may cry, you may feel anger and there is no shame in either, but you will also find courage and beauty and love in the process.

In industrial societies such as ours the major causes of death are heart disease and cancer. The majority of people die in an institution, e.g. a hospital or nursing home, but many die at home.

Shift from hospital to home care: The role of the team

Increasingly the patient's right to choose where he will die is being recognised and respected. The District Nurse must work particularly closely with the other members of the Primary Health Care Team in order to provide the best possible care for the patient dying at home.

Most patients prefer to die at home if adequate resources and support are available. This multidisciplinary and interdisciplinary approach gives the patients and family what they need where they want it.

E. R. Hillier (1983)

The recognition of the particular needs of the terminally ill has led to a rapid development in specialist services (since 1975). The growth of the hospice movement has demonstrated the value of 'care not cure' orientated institutions with emphasis on symptom control.

It is important that this expertise is sought and acted on by all health workers involved in the care of the terminally ill thus ensuring that home care is in no way inferior to that provided in institutions.

Home support teams attached to a hospice or hospital give care and advice not only to the dying patient and his family (Fig. 7.1) but equally provide the same expertise and support to District Nurses.

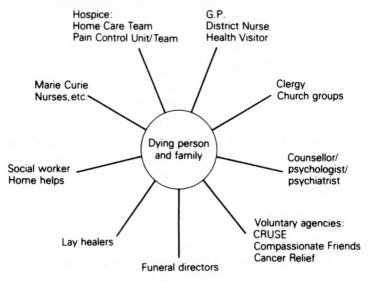

Fig. 7.1   Care of the dying and bereaved: the team

Inpatient vs. home care: The comparison of inpatient and out-patient care shows that both methods can be effective. Patients gave most praise to the outpatient system of care despite experiencing a little anxiety or irritability at home. J. Hinton (1979).

Cancer is a word not a sentence

Despite the increasingly good results from the treatment of cancer, cancer is still one of the most feared and dreaded diagnoses and people dying of cancer are stigmatised by others and often feel ashamed and terrified themselves. People dying of other diseases do not evoke the same sense of failure on the part of medical and nursing staff nor the same terror and distaste from the general public. This chapter concentrates therefore on the needs of patients dying of cancer, many of whom are cared for at home.

Alice's story

When they first told me I had it in my leg, I thought 'Oh well, I'll have whatever treatment is necessary; I'll fight it, and that'll be the end of it.' I was naturally fed up when they told me I'd have to have my leg off, but I thought 'Well after this I'll have beaten it.'

So I had my leg off and I adapted well. I got an automatic car and learnt how to drive. I changed my lifestyle. I couldn't go camping or walking any more, that was a bit of a disappointment, but I got over it.

Then it went to the lungs. I was so annoyed. I'd been through all that and it had come back. Well, I had chemotherapy and hoped that would be the end of it. Well, then I found this lump in my abdomen. I must admit that drained me. I get down now because I keep feeling all these lumps in my stomach. I had radiotherapy, but it didn't seem to do much. So I knew then. I don't think I've got much fight left in me now though. I feel too tired. It's all gone.

Facing our own feelings: staff stress

'Acknowledging a common humanity which includes at times feelings of inadequacy and anxiety, and talking over problems with colleagues is a sign of growth, not weakness.'

J. Robbins (1983)

District Nurses spend only approximately 10% of their work time with the terminally ill (Dunnel, K. & Dobbs, J., 1982). They do not usually experience the high stress levels their colleagues in cancer hospitals or in the hospices have to cope with. There are times, however, when a District Nurse may have been very close to the family, giving support, or have a 'run of deaths' or unusually large numbers of terminally ill patients in her care (and, as noted previously, in the future more people will die at home), and it is important therefore that all District Nurses recognise the warning signs of their own stress, e.g. fatigue, anxiety or apathy, and have ways of dealing with it. For example, talk to colleagues about it, set time aside for life affirming activities such as dancing, being with the children, or consider a change of job.

Some problems faced by the dying and the nurse's role

The dying patient and his family will face numerous problems, some may be insoluble but the majority might be easily overcome by medical and nursing care.

Problems faced by the dying

- communication problems
- direct effects of the disease and treatment
- unassociated physical symptoms or disease
- adjustment reactions to enforced changes in role
- pre-existing social and psychological problems

Adapted from: A. Stedeford (1984)

Communication problems

Does he know? Should he be told? This is a question many nurses worry about when learning to care for dying patients. Studies of such patients have shown that the majority – 95% in one sample (J. Hinton, 1967) – were well aware of their situation even without being told, although some were reluctant to talk about it with their family.

Case histories

John, a 49 year old printer, suffered from severe backache. Tests showed a primary carcinoma of the lung with metastases in the bones. John lives with his 45 year old wife and three young teenage children. Although his wife and the children know that John is dying, they believe him to be totally unaware of his diagnosis and prognosis ('He thinks he's got arthritis'). By insisting that John is not told the truth, his wife maintains that she is allowing him to enjoy the brief time left. The fact is, however, that he is probably fully aware of his situation. He confided to the District Nurse, 'I know something else is the matter, more serious than arthritis, maybe cancer. I'm so tired – I'm not getting better, I can't even wash myself. My younger child avoids me – cries all the time because "Daddy is ill" – I'm scared about the future. I'm scared about the pain. But I can't talk about it to my wife. She thinks she's protecting me but she's protecting herself as well, she can't face up to reality.'

By allowing John to talk about his anxieties and honestly answering his questions the District Nurse was able to assure John that his pain could be controlled and his fears contained. The decision not to discuss his condition with his wife was respected and he died with his wife still believing that he thought he had arthritis.

Different families and patients cope with the matter of a dying member differently. Some wish to maintain a facade to the end. It maybe necessary for the well-being of the whole family for the nurse to collude in this. Even when both partners have been told what the position is they may chose to deny it.

Mr & Mrs Brown, for example, were in their 70's. They had been told that Mrs Brown had cancer of the breast and needed surgery and radiotherapy. Mrs Brown refused to go to hospital and denies that she has cancer. She will not talk about her breast lesion or look at the dressing. Her husband, who hates to see his wife upset, also denies her illness and the fact that she is dying. Many people, however, want to know what is wrong and whether they are dying.

As one young woman patient called Alice put it, 'Some people just have to be told, don't they? I was one of them. I just had to know what I was up against, what I had to fight – and I fought all the way.'

The role of the District Nurse is *not* to insist on telling the patient 'the truth' or denying it – it is to provide ample opportunity for the patient to ask questions and to answer them tactfully and honestly. Where the family adamantly refuse to allow the dying person to be told what is wrong, it is best to set aside the time to talk to them privately, allowing them to express their feelings on the matter. Explain to them that their relative may well suffer more from fear of the unknown than from an honest explanation of his position, which almost certainly they have realised already.

Here again discussion of the problem and what has been said with the other members of the Primary Health Care Team, especially the G.P., is essential to avoid confused or contradictory information being given to the patient and his family.

At no point, however, should a 'time of death' be given to either the patient or the family – it is almost impossible for anyone to tell how long the final phase of life may last and saying 'one week' or 'two months', only produces unhappy results, particularly when the timetable proves incorrect and the patient continues to live past the date given. A space must always be left for hope.

As a general rule it is right to let the patient control the flow of information, and to assume that if he does not make use of good opportunities to ask questions, he should not be confronted with the seriousness of his condition.

A. Stedeford (1984)

Pain

Most patients, their families and indeed the general public believe that terminal illness (particularly as a result of cancer) is always accompanied by intense and possibly unrelievable pain. This is not true!

> As many as half of all patients with terminal cancer have no pain, or negligible discomfort at most. Forty per cent experience severe pain and the remaining ten per cent suffer less intense pain. Furthermore it is theoretically possible to relieve the pain in every case.
>
> R. G. Twycross (1975)

It is important to remember that not all pain in people with advanced cancer is necessarily due to the process of the disease. A patient dying of cancer is still, as much as any of us, liable to toothache, peptic ulcers, arthritis, cystitis or ingrowing toenails, and the pain from these 'minor' conditions may be the most important problem for the patient. It is therefore essential that a correct diagnosis of the cause of the pain is made to enable appropriate treatment to be given (e.g. removal of a rotten tooth, antibiotics and fluids for cystitis, etc.). Pain may be described as a complex 'mind–body' experience because it is impossible to separate the experience of mental from physical pain. All chronic pain therefore has social, psychological and physical aspects, and any treatment must be directed at all three. Dealing with the physical pain (e.g. by chemotherapy) will not necessarily remove the experience of pain if the patient is suffering anxiety, depression or social isolation. There is much the District Nurse can do to relieve pain at all three levels.

> Patients do not overrate their pain, certainly not when we have been able to gain their confidence. Most important though is that we *hear what they are trying to say*.
>
> C. Saunders (1983)

Assessment

As noted earlier pain is not a separate entity but part and parcel of the individual's total experience. It is therefore necessary that the assessment of pain should be seen as *part of the District Nurse's usual total patient assessment* in conjunction with the doctor's assessment and any additional information from other members of the Primary Health Care Team, hospital and/or hospice. *Non-verbal cues (e.g. hand and facial expressions) are as important as verbal ones.* Remember the pain may be due to:

1   The process of the cancer or past therapy
2   Unrelated physical problems or disease
3   Psycho-social factors

Factors affecting pain threshold:

Threshold lowered	Threshold raised
discomfort/pain	relief of symptoms
sleeplessness	sleep
fatigue	rest
anxiety	sympathy
fear	understanding
anger	companionship
sadness	diversional activity
depression	reduction in anxiety
boredom	elevation of mood
introversion	drugs e.g. analgesics
mental isolation	reduce loneliness
social abandonment	antidepressants

R. Twycross in Corr & Corr (1983)

Anything that raises the pain threshold reduces the experience of the pain, as can be seen from the list above. There are numerous strategies that the District Nurse can employ to raise the threshold over and above the correct administration of prescribed drugs:

Good basic nursing care will help reduce and prevent pain. Ensuring a *well aired, clean and pleasing environment* without imposing standards on the patient and family that are at odds with their normal lifestyle. A foul-smelling room reduces the likelihood of social contact for the patient.

Ensuring that the patient is comfortable; passive exercises and turning to prevent contractures and pressure sores, correct positioning especially when eating and drinking, gentle massage.

Maintaining the patient's personal appearance and self-esteem; hair, make-up, deodorants and mouth care are all important.

Ensuring that possible side effects from drugs and debility are noted and treated, particularly constipation, thrush in the mouth or vagina, cystitis, peptic ulcers, nausea and drowsiness and confusion.

Ensuring appropriate nutrition and fluid intake. The dying patient may well desire particular foods but when actually faced with them, feels unable to eat. The family should be assured that it is not necessary or kind to force the person to eat any more than he desires. Fluid intake should be encouraged for as long as possible. Ice lollies made of wine or fruit juice appeal to some people. Mouth cleaning with swabs is necessary and vital for comfort.

> Good nursing is the cornerstone of home care at the end of a patient's life and this in turn depends on imagination and effective symptom control, together with some knowledge of how to ease family distress.
>
> C. Saunders (1983)

Care plan for John

Problem: John complains of insomnia, due in part at least to the pain in his back.

Goal: To relieve the insomnia by achieving total pain control throughout the night and reducing any contributing factors, e.g. anxiety.

Nursing Care: Reassess John's pain (type, time, what aggravates or relieves it) frequently. Request the G.P. to visit to reassess the adequacy of the analgesia and ask about longer acting drugs or the addition of sedatives. Teach John and his family the principles of good pain relief management, and remove any misunderstandings about the fear of addiction. Encourage actions that might raise the pain threshold, e.g. listening to the radio or practising breathing exercises to maximise relaxation. Order a ripple bed to relieve the added discomfort of bedsores, and a backrest to aid comfortable positioning.

Provide counselling and support to reduce anxiety and fear regarding the process of the disease and associated pain as these can cause insomnia and lower the pain threshold.

Evaluation: When the pain history is taken, it reveals that John is trying to avoid taking pills until the pain is severe, which is about every 3 hours. The G.P. visited and prescribed long-acting pain tablets and a sedative to reduce his anxiety. John and family now understand the need to take the pills before the pain reappears. Practice relaxation and breathing exercises effectively. The ripple bed and back rest arrived and he uses them correctly. John is now sleeping through the night, i.e. from midnight to 7 a.m. and considers this satisfactory.

Analgesia in terminal care

It is the doctor's responsibility to prescribe the patient's medication; the District Nurse however must be vigilant in assessing the extent to which the prescription meets the patient's needs and to inform the doctor accordingly. It is not within the scope of this book to discuss the wide range of drugs available or their dosage. The general principles of analgesia are the same whatever the drug, and must be explained clearly to the patient and the family if compliance is to be obtained.

NB: Wherever possible frequent regular injections should be avoided in terminal care. People do not get used to intramuscular injections and the fear and dislike of them lowers the pain threshold. District Nurses should be aware of the current 'good practice' in relation to drugs and wherever an alternative to injections exists e.g. suppositories, tablets, liquid or syringe pumps, the doctor should be encouraged to prescribe the medication in that form.

The problems of unrelieved pain

Unlike the patient in hospital or hospice or nursing home, the patient dying at home is usually responsible, with his carers, for administering their own analgesia (unless it is by injection). Although this has advantages for the patient, allowing him some sense of control and participation in his care, it may equally cause problems. An inadequate understanding of the principles of administering analgesia for example, combined with poor communication between the family and the District Nurse or G.P. may well result in the patient suffering pain unnecessarily.

Dr Robert Wycross (1983) provides a check-list of common reasons for unrelieved pain resulting from this situation.

Reasons for unrelieved pain: check-list
1   Patient believes that pain is inevitable and untreatable.
2   Patient does not inform doctor or nurse, or puts on 'a brave face'.
3   Patient does not accept or take the medication as prescribed because he does not understand the principles of analgesia e.g.:
- Believes medication should only be taken if absolutely necessary
- Fears 'addiction'
- Fears that he will become 'tolerant' and nothing will be left for when 'things get really bad'

4   Stops medication because of unpleasant side effects but doesn't tell doctor or nurse because he fears they will disapprove

Patient teaching

If unrelieved pain due to such causes is to be avoided, it is vital that the District Nurse provide adequate and effective teaching for the family on all aspects of pain and its relief, the correct administration of drugs, what to expect and what to do about any possible side effects.

Unfortunately unrelieved pain may also be the result of the G.P.'s inappropriate treatment. Some doctors may, as Twycross (1983) points out, ignore the patient's pain because he believes it to be inevitable or intractable. He may not appreciate the intensity of the pain – accepting the patient's brave assertions that, 'I'm all right, doctor', and therefore prescribes inadequate analgesia or analgesia to be taken PRN (as required). Doctors, like patients, may inappropriately fear addiction and hold potent drugs in reserve for when the patient is 'really terminal'. Due to lack of knowledge doctors may be unaware of the required dosage of drugs for use in terminal care or the use of additional non-narcotic drugs as adjunctive therapy.

In these circumstances the nurse is in a very delicate position. Her obligation is to act as her patient's advocate and she must use all her tact to ensure her patient's needs for pain relief are met. It may be necessary to seek advice and support from her supervisors, colleagues and the expertise of the hospice care team or specialist nurse adviser on how to best achieve this objective.

> It is the duty of every District Nurse not to give in to a dismissive general practitioner until she has obtained relief for her patient.
>
> H. Copperman (1983)

Signs of approaching death

Very few people in our society have ever seen a dead person – even fewer have watched someone die. Screaming terrified people fighting for life or blood pouring forth from the dying person's body are the images of the last hours of life that many people hold. One of the most important things the District Nurse can do is to assure both patient and carers that death is very rarely an unpleasant experience. One can in all honesty say that usually people become increasingly tired and eventually drift into unconsciousness and sleep. The last moments when the body dies are tranquil.

The family may want to know how they will recognise that the patient is approaching death and how they can help to comfort their loved one at this time. Some signs of approaching death and suggestions for care are given below. Both family and nurses who have never witnessed a death often fear that they will not recognise that the person is dead – but this is rarely the case.

Death itself is usually not so much an event as an absence of presence when the spirit of the person has ceased or departed. The heartbeat and breathing stops. The body appears relaxed and the face is usually calm.

Approaching death signs:

Withdrawal from social interaction; feels very tired	Allow the patient to be quiet – remain with him but do not force him to talk or participate in family life. Allow him 'personal space' and time to think.
Becomes restless and drowsy and agitated; may pluck at the bedclothes	Continue to give pain relief – gentle massage may comfort him. Agitation may be due to constipation and/or retention of urine. A catheter may be appropriate. Drugs may be given.
Refuses or dislikes taking food or drink; too weak to eat	Do not force food or drink, but offer small pieces of fruit or ice. Keep mouth moist and clean with ice chips, mouth swabs soaked in water or mouthwash. Put cream on lips to avoid cracking.
Skin colour changes (pallor, cyanosis and/or jaundice)	Maintain skin care and turning if patient is not too disturbed by this.
Pulse becomes weak, rapid and/or irregular; wrist pulse may be undetectable.	
Changes in breathing – noisy 'rattle' due to secretions in throat, gasping for air, possible internal bleeding, Cheyne	This can be particularly worrying to family – fear of the 'death rattle' or 'Cheyne Stokes'. Drugs may be prescribed to dry

Stokes and stops then cycle repeats until death

secretions or a change of position may help.

Eyes may become glazed, may remain open or unconscious, fixed stare.

Family may find this very disturbing. Keep eyes clean and moist.

Incontinence of urine and/or faeces due to relaxation of sphincters

Upsetting for everyone – maintain patient's hygiene using deodorants as necessary.

Increasing coldness of body, especially limbs; cold sweating.

Massage of feet and hands may comfort. Bathe face and keep skin dry. Maintain warm but keep covers off the body. Use a bed cradle as every cover feels heavy.

Changing level of consciousness; may appear comatose then regain awareness then sink into coma again. Coma usually precedes death. Patient appears calm and at rest.

Encourage family to remain with patient explaining that the sense of hearing remains to the end, so gentle conversation or prayer may be welcome. Holding the patient gently, but not clinging on to him is comforting for everyone.

Adapted from J. Robbins (1983)

The patient's reactions to impending death

The way a person approaches death is as unique as the way he lives; it is part of life. Certain patterns of response however can be anticipated which dying patients typically pass through. Dr Kubler Ross (1982) identified five such stages but it is important to realise that not every person will go through each stage and that some people who, for example, have reached 'acceptance', may at a later point in their illness return to a state of 'denial' or 'anger'.

Kubler Ross – Stages of dying and nurse's response:

Denial:
It can't be true

Allow patient to control information; provide information when asked. Listen and provide support.

Anger: Why me . . . ?	Do not take attacks personally, empathise; explain the 'normality' of this stage to family; let him express his anger and irritation.
Bargaining: It's me *but* . . .	Usually this is a private response; if it becomes public, show understanding
Depression: Yes . . . me	Allow person to grieve and mourn openly; drug treatment *may be considered appropriate,* discuss with doctor.
Acceptance: Anxiety gone, unfinished business is completed.	Allow patient to be calm and detached; continue to be supportive.

Families' reactions to a member's impending death

The members of the family will also experience some of the stages outlined above. The time it takes different individuals to work through these stages varies; consequently the patient may well reach the stage of acceptance while his spouse is still at the denial or depressed stage. Alice, for example (quoted earlier), knew, as she put it, 'what she was up against'; she had reached some point of acceptance having 'fought all the way'. Her husband, Peter, on the other hand is still at the denial stage.

Their daughter said of him, 'He doesn't cope with the fact that she's dying at all. He just doesn't accept it. He hides from it, he won't face up to it. He won't talk about it because he just doesn't believe it, even though he's been told.'

Bereavement care

From the moment when the family have been told that their loved one is terminally ill the process of grieving begins. This anticipatory grief is part of the necessary process of coming to terms with loss. It can sometimes, however, be counterproductive and add to the dying patient's sense of isolation. This is particularly so when the family have been told that he will only live a specific time (e.g. three months); if the patient in fact continues to live past this time, the family may have completed the grieving process and feel a sense of distance from the loved one during their last weeks. This emphasises the need to avoid any definite statements concerning the length of time remaining to any patient. The nurse's role is to support the family during this phase of grief while enabling them and their loved one to live fully until he dies.

> 'In the jungles of Mexico one custom after someone dies is that each person who comes to the burial or to visit asks the mourner to recount the story of how the death happened. The visitors probably already know, but the point is to keep the mourner repeating and repeating the story until the shock lessens and he or she begins to accept what's happened. . . . Listen and listen and listen.'
>
> D. Duda (1982)

After the death

Following the patient's death the grief process continues and intensifies. The actual grief reaction or behaviour will differ markedly from one person to another. It will depend on a number of factors – the bereaved's own personality, previous experience of loss, relationship with the patient, age of the patient, length of the patient's illness, how he died and the family's cultural traditions and religious beliefs.

It is, however, possible to outline the process or tasks of mourning most bereaved people will experience.

Four tasks of mourning:

1   To accept the reality of the loss.
Many people deny – at some level – that their loved one has died – they feel he is away on business or abroad.
2   To experience the pain of grief.
In some cultures – notably our own – people may feel they need to be brave and not allow themselves to feel the pain of their loss.
3   To adjust to an environment in which the deceased is missing.
This is not just the loss of a loved one, but usually involves the loss of status for the survivor and the loss of the roles and services performed by the loved one.
4   To withdraw emotional energy and to reinvest it in another relationship.
This may be seen as a betrayal of the deceased or a decision never again to risk experiencing the pain of loss.

Source: J. W. Worden (1983)

Goals of grief/bereavement counselling:

The overall goal is to help the survivor complete any unfinished business with the deceased and be able to say a final goodbye. The specific goals are:

1   To increase the reality of the loss
2   To help the survivor deal with both expressed and latent effects of the loss
3   To help overcome various impediments to readjustment after the loss
4   To encourage a healthy emotional withdrawal from the deceased and to feel comfortable reinvesting that emotion in another relationship.

Adapted from : J. W. Worden (1983)

What to do when someone dies

Where death has been anticipated there is no question of heroic attempts at resuscitation. The minutes following death should be a time of calmness, not action. Time for the nurse to gather her thoughts, bid farewell to the patient and support the family. The nurse should simply straighten the body, clean away any blood, etc., gently close the eyes if they have remained open. It is not necessary to do 'last offices' in the patient's home – nor is it desirable to cover the person's face or hands. The relatives should be encouraged to sit by the body and say their own farewell. They may be frightened to touch the body but a quiet word from the nurse should make it clear that it is perfectly acceptable to hold their loved one's hand or kiss them. It is tactful to absent oneself for a time so that the family can be alone – making a cup of tea is usually appreciated. The nurse may be asked to inform the doctor and undertaker that the patient has died and the exact time of death. The family may well ask the District Nurse what has to be done in the time following death.

It is important to remember that we live in a culturally mixed society and at times like birth and death people cling to their traditions. If the family are Moslems, Hindus or Jews they may not wish their relative's body to be touched by someone of another faith and the nurse must, therefore, ask permission before handling the body to avoid causing further distress to the relatives.

Before leaving always allow time to listen to any fears or feelings of guilt they may have. A few words of praise for the care they have given and an assurance that you will come back to talk again at a later time is a kindness that will long be remembered.

What must be done when the patient dies:

Different religions and cultures will have particular forms of mourning and funeral arrangements. But some actions are required by all people in the UK.
1   Inform the *doctor* that the death has occurred.
2   If the doctor has not seen the patient within the past fortnight the

coroner is informed.

3   Doctor issues a Certificate of Death. If the patient is to be *cremated* he will arrange for a second doctor to sign.

4   Inform *family* and *friends* and *clergy*.

5   Contact *undertaker* – they will remove the body or leave it in the house as the family wish. They will advise the family about funeral costs and arrangements.

6   The death must be registered at the local office of the *Registrar of Births, Marriages and Deaths* within 5 days. A relative or friend can do this. He issues a Certificate of Disposal and a Certificate of Registration of Death.

7   A *Death Grant* (£15–£30) can be claimed from the Social Security Office The Death Certificate and an estimate of funeral costs must be taken when making the claim. Leaflet N149 gives further information about extra financial assistance that may be obtainable.

The right to die?

Assisted suicide or mercy killing, i.e. euthanasia, is illegal in Britain. The rights or wrongs of euthanasia are, however, increasingly discussed both publicly on television programmes and privately, particularly by families with a dying member. It is important therefore for the District Nurse to be informed on and to have considered the issues involved although clearly she should at no time encourage or support any action of this sort. Reassurance to both patient and family that death and dying can be pain free and distressing symptoms controlled will allay much of the anxiety and fear that lead people to contemplate facilitating their loved one's death prematurely.

Test yourself

1   What problems are faced by the dying person?
2   Should a dying person be told?
3   In what ways may the District Nurse help to relieve pain?
4   What are the signs of approaching death?
5   What must be done when a patient dies?
6   What are the tasks of mourning?
7   What experience of loss have you had? How did you cope with the feeling?
8   Can euthanasia ever be condoned?

8 The role of the District Nurse in the care of the chronically sick person and family

One of the consequences of the improvement in medicine, drugs and environmental health is that many people who would in the past have died of their disease or intercurrent infection now survive, often for many years. Chronic illnesses managed in the community by the District Nurse and other members of the Primary Health Care Team include multiple sclerosis, arthritis, stroke, chronic bronchitis and emphysema, heart disease, cancer, diabetes, mental illness and senile dementia and varicose ulcers.

The District Nurse's work is almost entirely concerned with the management of chronic illness. Table 8.1 shows the percentage of time spent on various conditions.

Shafer *et al.* (1979) describe chronic illness as one caused by disease that produces symptoms and signs within a variable period of time, that runs a long course and from which there is only partial recovery . . . a chronic illness is characterised by remissions and exacerbations

Table 8.1 Time spent managing chronic illness.

Condition	Percentage of District Nurse's time
Postoperation hospital discharge	7
Terminal/deteriorating	9
Physical handicap	27
Mental handicap/illness	4
Chest disease	3
Cardiovascular disease	11
Skin, sores and ulcers	13
Diabetic	7

Adapted from: Dunnell, K. & Dobbs, J. (1982)

and slowly progressive physical changes (Fig. 8.1).

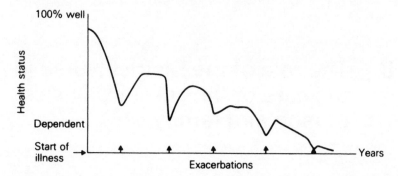

Fig. 8.1   Health profile of a patient with chronic illness

Chronic illness is usually experienced as an impaired function of a number of the body's systems. It has not only long-term physical but also long-term psychological, social and spiritual consequences. Indeed the demands made by the illness affect and/or disrupt every aspect of the patient's and carer's life and can never be eliminated or forgotten.

The patient with Multiple Sclerosis for example is faced with boredom, decreased social skills, family strains, physical deterioration and a negative self-image. For that individual there is no escape. Social relationships are disrupted and even disintegrate under the impact of reduced mobility, speech difficulties and lack of symptom control. The sufferer becomes socially isolated, by those who cannot face the physically altered person they once knew, nor the embarrassment of visiting.

Despite individual differences and the varying progress of particular chronic diseases, one aspect common to all these patients is the feeling that they are losing or have lost control over their own life, i.e. they feel powerless.

Factors leading to a sense of powerlessness:

1   The unpredictable progress of the disease process
2   Failure of therapy to provide a cure
3   Physical deterioration despite sticking to the prescribed regime, increasing fatigue
4   Side effects of treatment
5   Reduction in patient's psychological stamina
6   Breakdown in support network, strain on carers
7   Fear for the future and its increased dependency
8   Uncertainty in all areas of the patient's life

Adapted from: Fitzgerald Miller, J. (1983)

Although specific treatments may be necessary in the case of chronic illness this is usually subordinate to more general nursing measures necessary to:

1   strengthen the individual and family's ability to function i.e. cope
2   encourage health-maximising behaviour
3   reduce and manage stress and
4   deal with fatigue

The priority in nursing the chronically ill person is, however, to enable the patient to feel as much in control of their life as possible. There are a number of ways in which the District Nurse can help to achieve this objective. Once again, however, this requires full use of the resources of the Primary Health Care Team members and their associates (e.g. the hospital, rehabilitation centre, etc.) can offer.

Some ways of maximising patient's sense of control

Modifying the environment. Any adaptations to the home e.g. ramp for wheelchair, low level kitchen, bath rails, etc. that enable the person some degree of independence are important. Arrange bedroom furniture and equipment to encourage self-care. Provide necessary aids e.g. walking frame.

Encouraging control over when and who visits – this must include the District Nurse and other helpers. Although it is often difficult for the District Nurse to make a specific appointment to visit a patient, he should be consulted and his wishes complied with as far as is possible. It is important to maximise areas of certainty, so if a visit is delayed the patient should be informed.

Knowledge is power: chronically ill people particularly need information about their illness and its management so that they can make decisions and take action relative to their condition and their future. Wherever possible the patient should be responsible for their own medication, etc. Explain where and how to get any additional information necessary.

Encourage the patient to express his feelings especially in relation to 'powerlessness' if it is appropriate. Identifying contributing factors and getting supportive feedback from the District Nurse increases his sense of control. The District Nurse will equally try to sensitise the carers to the patient's feelings and vice versa.

Setting realistic goals. The patient should participate in devising his care plan and setting *realistic* goals. Success breeds success and by reaching a self-care goal, however limited, the patient's sense of control is increased. It may be making telephone contact with a self-help group or washing one's own hands. Goals should be short-term to enable progress to be easily observed.

Encourage health-maximising behaviour within the limits imposed by the disease. Maintain maximum mobility through exercise. Ensure correct positioning to avoid pressure sores. Encourage adequate rest to avoid fatigue. Promote the use of relaxation techniques. Emphasise the need to eat a healthy diet and drink sufficient fluids. Anticipate and treat any further complications or illness. Avoid accidents by taking precautions. Provide opportunities for self-expression and growth. Support any evidence of pride in appearance.

Minimise any undesirable side effects of the condition. Any person in a dirty or offensive smelling environment experiences a loss of self-esteem. Fear of 'smelling bad' or looking ill kempt will reduce the patient's sense of confidence and control.

The role of the Primary Health Care Team and its associates in the care of chronically ill patients and families is summarised in Fig. 8.2.

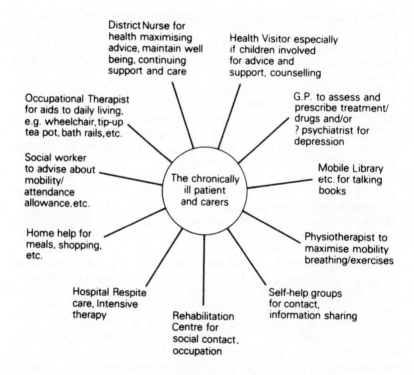

Fig. 8.2   The role of the Primary Health Care Team and associates

Coping strategies of the chronically ill and their carers

Hope. Although the District Nurse is committed to providing the patient and family with a realistic assessment of their situation, this does not and should not destroy hope. On the contrary the ability to hope whatever the circumstances is a powerful human resource. Hope means looking forward to living as fully as possible – not necessarily to a complete cure. The nurse encourages positive thoughts such as, 'I can do it, they may find a new drug – I'm better off than many', and discourages negative statements that decrease self-esteem, e.g. 'I'm useless.'

Concealment of the illness and its effects – as far as is possible. Everyone wants to appear normal and especially during a period of remission the chronically ill patient and his family will go to great lengths to conform to 'normality'. The District Nurse can help to devise such strategies e.g. a leg bag and advise on deodorants, or give a map with all the public toilets marked.

The dangers of this strategy are that the effort involved in maintaining 'normality' may be very draining, and that it may encourage the family and patient to reject help or services because 'the neighbours will realise something is wrong', e.g. incontinent laundry service.

Pacing, i.e. identifying what one can do and how long it will take. Both the patient and carer are experts in this subject. The District Nurse will support this strategy as it enables the patient to remain in control and independent for as long as possible.

Rehabilitation/adaptation in chronic illness

Rehabilitation of the chronically ill person if defined narrowly as 'returning the individual to full functioning' is clearly not an appropriate aim. It is more accurate to describe it as 'positive adaptation to a changed physical, psychological and social situation'. One writer considers it as 'coming to terms existentially with the reality of chronic illness as a state of being, discarding both false hope and destructive hopelessness, restructuring the environment in which one must now function' (Feldman, 1974).

The chronically ill patient (and his family) have experienced a significant loss – indeed a series of losses – like the bereaved or dying person they need time and support to work through their grief to a point of acceptance of the changed circumstances. Only after this stage is reached can positive adaptation take place.

Losses of the chronically ill:

- of health and functions: energy – strength and vitality, ability to communicate verbally, muscle co-ordination, bowel and bladder control
- of body parts/positive body image: organs, hair, weight
- of roles: breadwinner, decision maker
- of a secure future: loss of predictability
- of self-esteem: dignity and privacy
- of intimacy: e.g. sexual closeness
- of relationships: no contact with friends
- of independence: inability for self-care
- of finance

Adapted from J. Fitzgerald Miller (1983)

Case history

Fifteen years ago Jenny Carstairs was told she had Multiple Sclerosis. She was thirty years old. The disease had an insidious onset and Jenny was not greatly incapacitated at first. Her husband, a high spirited businessman, supported her through this change and they often went out together. However, tragically he died five years later. Since that time Jenny's problems have increased – she also had a car crash which brought on a marked deterioration in her physical condition.

Her mother, Mrs Ford, moved in to take care of Jenny. Jenny began to spend most of her time in bed, which was not warranted by the pathological stage of her illness; in fact she could do most things by herself. Mrs Ford was sorry for Jenny and lavished attention on her. Jenny, however, resented her mother's 'takeover'. She was aggressive and demanding and showed no signs of appreciating her mother's help – indeed she felt her mother was contributing to her incapacity. Nevertheless she continued to remain weak and passive rather than risk losing the attention she was receiving. As time passed Mrs Ford grew increasingly angry at Jenny's refusal to do anything to help herself. The mutual hostility engendered ended with Mrs Ford returning to her own home leaving Jenny in a very difficult situation, especially as she had treated the G.P. and social worker and the District Nurse in the same abusive manner. Mrs Ford, overcome with guilt, returned a few months later.

This history highlights some of the tension between patient and carer or District Nurse when trying to encourage adaptation (Fig. 8.3).

The warning signs of stress will be monitored by the District Nurse. Such signs include:

1   An increasing sense of fatigue – greater than would be expected in relation to work done.

2   Irritability with the patient or other people.
3   Anxiety over small things, over conscientious.
4   Frequent minor illness e.g. headaches, insomnia.
5   Feelings of depression and apathy
6   Increasing use of alcohol, tobacco and/or drugs.

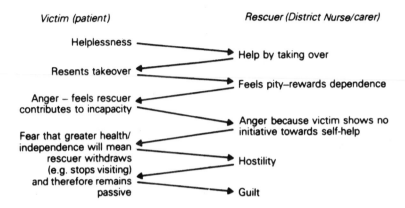

Fig. 8.3   Problems of encouraging adaption/rehabilitation when caring for the chronically sick: the Rescue Game

Strength – the family's ability to function and cope and deal with fatigue

'I never get out. It's hard work. He can't get out of bed even to use the commode. I have to sleep down here on the settee – I have done ever since the first stroke. If I'm not here he may try and get up and fall. I just lie here and watch what he's doing through the chairs . . . I don't sleep much, because it's not very comfortable. We've had a solid three years of it and the last year has been the worst.'

Fatigue – especially associated with sleep disturbance – is the major problem carers of the chronically ill experience – as indeed do the patients. The District Nurse encourages the carer to take adequate rest by enlisting extra help, e.g. other relatives, who may take on some of the burden of care. A home help will provide some time in which the carer can rest. Realistically, however, the carer often finds it psychologically impossible to rest while the patient is at home and for this reason the District Nurse may arrange some form of day care or a 'Respite Stay' in hospital.

Case history

Understand stress in the family – interpersonal relations, e.g. disruption of children's lives:

Jenny, a widow, has two children. She accused her mother of spoiling them. Her daughter, Susan (15 years old) began to behave very badly, was expelled from school, and spent a lot of time with a rough gang of older boys. She was sent away to boarding school. Her son, Tim (12 years old), became quieter and withdrawn and was doing badly in his class.

In this case the District Nurse asked the social worker who knew Jenny to give the children long-term support. She advised Jenny and her mother what to do to minimise the damage the disruption of Jenny's illness and their father's death had clearly had on Tim and Susan.

We have already noted the difficult relationship between Jenny and her mother. The District Nurse assists in this situation by remaining impartial but acting as an advocate or middleman to encourage open recognition of the problem. Once identified and explained, problems can be more easily managed.

A long discussion which provides opportunities for the carers to express their feelings to a supportive listener will go some way towards reducing stress. Providing practical assistance to reduce the work load and allow the carers some free time is also important. In some cases it may be necessary for the District Nurse to refer the carer to the G.P. for some drug therapy to see them over the crisis – though this is rarely the best solution. Particular underlying causes of stress e.g. financial worries should be dealt with by an appropriate referral to the social worker.

Test yourself

1   What characterises a chronic illness?
2   What factors may lead to a feeling of 'powerlessness'?
3   How can the District Nurse help to reduce feelings of 'powerlessness'?
4   What problems may the carer experience when looking after a chronically ill person?
5   What facilities are available in your area to relieve the burden on the carer?

9 The role of the District Nurse in promoting continence

Prevalence of urinary incontinence: the iceberg phenomenon

While out with the District Nurse you will visit many people who have problems with maintaining continence. You may well assume that the majority of incontinent people are under the care of a District Nurse. This is far from the case.

Incidence of regular incontinence in the community

Age	Male Percentage	Female Percentage
5–14	6.9	5.1
15–64	1.6 (0.1)	11.6 (0.2)
65+	6.9 (1.3)	11.6 (2.5)

Number in brackets = people known to be incontinent by health or social service workers.

Source: T. Thomas *et al.* (1980)

The iceberg phenomenon: We are only seeing the tip of the iceberg of the problem of incontinence in the community.

What is incontinence?

Voiding in the wrong place and in a way that undermines self-esteem. The cause may be physical, psychological, environmental. It may be reversible or irreversible. It is a symptom not a disease which can sometimes be cured, can often be improved and can always be more easily managed.

Incontinence is concealed for as long as feasible, if possible for ever. Many people, particularly women, are believed to be unable to discuss it, even with their doctor.

District Nurses therefore have an important **health education role** in relation to continence promotion:

- In the wider community by disseminating information and reducing the taboo of incontinence
- With families where a member is known to be incontinent but it is hidden from health care professionals
- With the incontinent patient and his carers

The elderly incontinent individual. The elderly are the major patient group of District Nurses and frequently suffer incontinence, though it affects all age groups, men and women equally, and has numerous underlying causes.

G.P. assessment and diagnosis. All incontinent patients require a medical examination to exclude or establish any underlying pathology or inappropriate medication. The District Nurse will therefore request a visit by the G.P. to assess the patient's medical condition. The long-term management however is the nurse's responsibility and the care of incontinent patients forms a major component of the District Nurse's work.

Types of incontinence

Stress: is the symptom of leaking urine coincidentally with physical exertion, such as coughing, laughing and lifting. Usually associated with a weakness or incompetence of the urethral sphincter mechanism and/or weakness in the muscles of the pelvic floor. Exacerbated by cough, obesity or constipation.

Urge: is the symptom of having to hurry to pass urine and is commonly due to bladder muscle instability and/or reduced nervous inhibition signal from the brain. Exacerbated by environmental factors, mobility problems and anxiety.

Dribble: is the symptom of having difficulty voiding urine, may be due to atonic bladder or outflow obstruction, e.g. enlarged prostate, leading to retention with overflow. Exacerbated by constipation.

Reflex: is the symptom of losing conscious control of the bladder through disease or injury, e.g. spinal injury. The bladder fills until contraction of the bladder muscle is stimulated via a nervous reflex arc. A baby's bladder empties in this way.

Passive: is the wetting at rest for no apparent reason. Possible physical causes are any of the above. Mental impairment e.g. dementia, confusion etc. Exacerbated by disorientation, physical handicaps, carers being unaware of individual needs and motivation.

Causes of incontinence:

1 *Intrinsic factors* (i.e. physical and mental disability)
2 *Reversible incontinence*

Diuresis	(osmotic)	renal failure
		hyperglycaemia
		hypercalcaemia
	(drugs)	strong diuretics
		anticholinergics (retention with overflow)
		Ephedrine
		sedatives
Atrophy		atrophic urethritis
		vaginitis (urinary tract infection)
Mechanical		prostate
		faecal impaction
		pelvic tumour
		stone
		stress incontinence
Psychological		depression
		anxiety
Environmental		toilet too far away

3 *Irreversible incontinence*:
Post prostatectomy symptoms.
Inhibition lost over reflex contractions (from cortical
centre in the frontal lobe)
Spinal lesions (motor and sensory loss)
Sensation loss (peripheral and nerve lesions)

Source: M. K. Thompson in Mandalstam 1980

Case history

Eighty year old Mrs Harding lives in her own bungalow with her grandchildren, Jane, 19 years old, and Peter, 17, as their parents are dead. Jane and Peter are rarely at home and resent having to live with their grandmother. There is therefore a lot of animosity between them. Because of her arthritis Mrs Harding is finding it difficult to rise and reach the toilet without help (i.e. difficulty with locomotion).

When the District Nurse visited her for the first time, Mrs Harding had been alone since early morning. She was sitting in a low chair and had been incontinent of urine.

Mrs Harding's story is typical of many elderly incontinent patients living at home. As she told the District Nurse, 'Just lately my leg has got very weak so I really need help to get up off the chair. I've slowed down a lot. I can't hold my water and that worries me. It's got worse especially now because I can't get up if my granddaughter isn't here. When she gets back home she grumbles at me for wetting – but I can't help it.

As with any patient a full assessment is essential. Before leaving the Health Centre the District Nurse will have already read all available notes and asked if any of her colleagues have already had contact with Mrs. Harding.

This process of information gathering continues on her journey to the patient's home – observing the area and noting its amenities. Even closer observation is called for on entering the home. She will use her ears and nose. Is it clean, warm, where is the toilet, does it smell? Listen to the conversation, what does it tell you about the family dynamics?

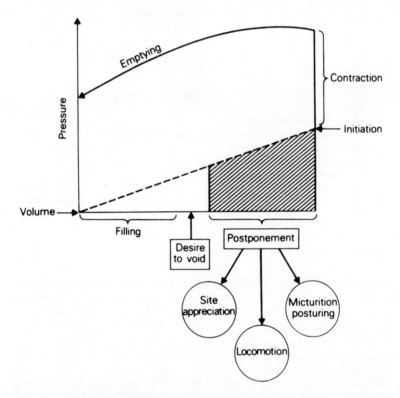

Fig. 9.1 Micturition Cycle: Filling up to the time of perceiving the desire to void. Voluntary postponement of the onset of micturition; identifying a place and circumstances where it is socially acceptable to urinate. *Possess mobility and dexterity to reach the place*, assume and maintain body posture during micturition – adjust clothing, deal with doors, locks, flushing system, get back to the starting point. *Source*: Yeates (1972)

Unlike hospital care the nursing of the patient in the community is dependent to a considerable extent on environmental factors in the patient's home and the surrounding area and even more importantly on the attitude and strengths of the people who are caring for the patient, e.g. daughter, granddaughter, neighbour, etc.

The first priority in relation to incontinent patients is to maintain and promote self-esteem. The District Nurse will help Mrs Harding wash and change into dry clothes. Remember however that even this will further undermine her as it emphasises her dependence on others to achieve this very basic activity of daily living. It must be done with the utmost tact!

When Mrs Harding is comfortable the District Nurse will start her assessment interview. This is best done in private. A relaxed, unhurried approach is essential – aided by a shared cup of tea.

Many old people minimise their difficulties for fear that they will be 'sent away' if they cause 'trouble'. The interview should reassure the patient that you want to help her achieve continence as far as possible and if this is not possible to improve the situation. The first step is to establish the cause of the incontinence and therefore a full history in conjunction with a doctor's diagnosis should be taken (including past and present illnesses, drug regime, especially when Mrs Harding actually takes her medicines and how much she takes). Over-sedation, or the taking of diuretics at the wrong time and bowel impaction are common causes of incontinence or it could be a very simple matter of not being able to reach the toilet. Dietary and fluid intake is particularly important.

Mrs Harding has reduced her fluid intake to a minimum in an attempt to reduce her urine output. She now has a urinary infection which has increased her incontinence (a specimen of urine for analysis should be taken if not already done by the G.P.).

The answers to the following questions indicate the reasons why the person is incontinent and should be part of your assessment (Coloplast Objective Continence, 1983):

Universal question: Is the person incontinent or just having problems maintaining continence, i.e. is it the primary problem, or is there an underlying cause?

What is the persons's complaint?
When did the accidents start?
Were they associated with any particular event?
Is the person taking any medication which could account for the incontinence (i.e. diuretics or night sedation)?
What is the result of urinalysis and rectal examination?
Is the person also wet at night?
Is the person drinking tea or coffee late at night?

Are toilet facilities nearby?
Would the person use a commode or urinal?
Are there mobility problems?
Are there low chair/cot sides or other barriers to mobility?
Could these be improved and improve continence?
Does the person have suitable aids? Specify.
Can the person communicate needs?
Is clothing a problem?
Is toilet routine frequent enough?
Is the person mentally alert and aware of the problem?
Is there any anxiety or depression?
Is the person denying the problem?
Has there been any recent emotional shock, such as a bereavement?
Is the problem affecting self-esteem and confidence?
Have you reassured the person?
Are social activities suffering?
Is the person's family under stress because of the problem?
What are the financial implications (e.g. buying of aids and washing)?
Can the person be taught pelvic floor exercises?
Is further examination needed?

Yes answers to the following questions could indicate:

Is the person not aware of bladder fullness? Is the leakage a continuous dribble?	Overflow incontinence, severe constipation, prostate problems
Is the leakage slight? Does it happen on exertion (e.g. coughing, laughing or sneezing)?	Stress incontinence, lax pelvic floor
Is the leakage great? Does the bladder empty without warning?	Reflex incontinence, unstable bladder
Does the person have a feeling of urgency? Does the person ever have accidents? How much warning time does the person get?	Urge incontinence, bladder irritability.

Remember: there may be more than one cause.

Three aspects of rehabilitation should be considered:

1 Means of maintaining continence (commode, urinals)
2 Means of retraining for continence, individualised toileting, bladder training, pelvic floor exercises
3 Means of containing incontinence (pads, pants, external appliances, catheters)

In Mrs Harding's case the design and layout of the environment added to her immobility and was the cause of her incontinence. The District Nurse must ask herself three questions (after Mandalstam, D., 1980):

1 *Can mobility be sufficiently improved to allow the person to reach the toilet in time?*

Is chiropody required?
Is there an underlying medical problem e.g. arthritis or Parkinson's disease which is slowing walking speed or making the person unsteady; are these conditions being dealt with adequately?
Would the person's mobility problems benefit from the advice of a physiotherapist e.g. by restoring confidence?
Are walking aids or rearrangement of furniture necessary?

2 *Can the journey to the toilet be made easier?*

Can the person be helped from the chair more quickly e.g. by better positioning of feet and placing hands correctly and moving to the edge of the chair?
Would a grab rail or bannister or stair-lift help?

3 *Can the toilet be brought nearer?*

Does the person have an inside toilet available (if not a local authority grant may be available)?
Does the toilet door need resiting to allow access?
Does the toilet seat need to be raised?
Would a commode be acceptable?
Would other urine collecting devices be advisable?

Planning care

Once the reason for incontinence has been determined, a care plan involving various steps can be undertaken to improve the situation (Fig. 9.2).

Together with Mrs Harding the rehabilitation plan is decided. This will include:

Charting the times of urination to establish a pattern and allow for appropriate toileting.
Teaching pelvic floor exercises and initiating bladder retraining.
Explaining the need for adequate fluid intake and regular bowel movements.
Reviewing the medicines prescribed and the best time to take them.
Discussing the use of a commode or walking appliance to effect more convenient toileting.
Pads and pants may be considered if the incontinence cannot be managed any other way.
Catheters should only be advised if incontinence is untreatable and this offers the best means of improving the patient's quality of life. (Intermittent self-catheterisation may be taught if appropriate.)

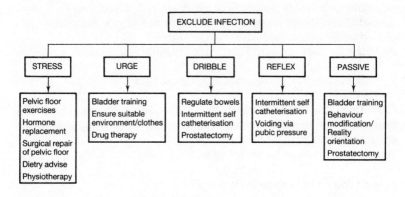

Fig. 9.2   Flowchart for the promotion of continence

Care plan for Mrs Harding

Problem: Mrs Harding is unable to reach the toilet in time.
Goal: To achieve continence by maximising mobility and increasing understanding of process of micturition (Fig. 9.1), for example the need for fluid intake.
Nursing care: Request chiropody, physiotherapy and G.P. visits. Order 'ejector' seat and commode. Teach and advise about the incontinence process and fluid intake requirements.

Evaluation: Chiropody, physiotherapy and G.P. visits suggest exercises and adjustment of medication. Mrs Harding used the new seat effectively and is able to reach commode alone thus being now continent.

Pelvic floor exercises

These exercises are most effective if carried out conscientiously over a period of at least six months. Improvement will be gradual so patience and perseverance are essential. These exercises are not just for women, men find that they have a beneficial effect as well.

Exercise 1: Sit, stand or lie comfortably, without tensing the muscles of the seat, abdomen or legs and pretend that you are trying to control diarrhoea by tightening the ring of muscle around the back passage. Do this several times until you feel certain that you have identified the area and are making the correct movement.

Exercise 2: Sit on the toilet or commode and commence to pass water, and whilst doing so, make an attempt to stop the flow in midstream by contracting the muscles around the front passage. Do this several times until you feel sure of the movement and the sensation of applying conscious control.

Exercise 3: Exercise as follows, sitting, standing or lying, tightening first the back passage muscles and then the front, and then do both together. Count four slowly, then release the muscles. Do this four times every hour if possible.

With practice the movements become easier to master and the exercises can be carried out at any time, such as waiting for a bus, ironing, watching TV or lying in bed.

Working with carers

It is very important that the District Nurse discusses the problem of incontinence and the proposed plan of action with not only the patients but with the carers. The success of any continence promotion will be as much determined by the willingness and abilities or otherwise of the carers to carry it out.

There is no point in formulating a nursing care plan unless it is with the agreement and support and within the capabilities of the patient and carer alike, which in Mrs Harding's case means the grandchildren. The District Nurse's persuasive and social skills are essential in encouraging and motivating Mrs Harding's grandchildren to co-operate in the planning and implementation of the continence promotion plan. The nurse acts on the patient's behalf explaining the condition and so reducing the stigma surrounding the patient.

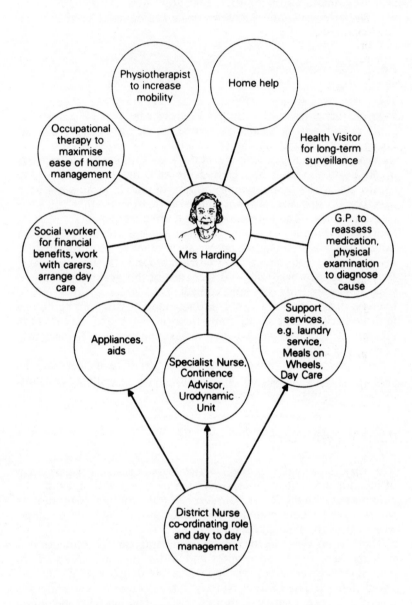

Fig. 9.3 The role of the Primary Health Care Team in the care of Mrs Harding

Incontinence: – The straw that breaks the camel's back:

> 'Studies have shown that incontinence is a major consideration in seeking nursing home places, 44% of relatives said this was a major factor, (Johnson & Werner study, 1982), 89% of elderly people themselves cited incontinence as a major reason.'
>
> (Smallegan 1985)

District Nurse is the co-ordinator of resources

Specialist advice: The particular expertise of the Specialist Nurse Continence Adviser, where available, will be sought and a joint visit arranged.

Support services: The District Nurse will organise the incontinence laundry service, disposal of soiled pads, Meals on Wheels, etc. and the assistance of a home help as appropriate.

Aids and appliances: Appliances, commodes, pads and pants, etc. are ordered if required.

Primary Health Care Team skills: The District Nurse will discuss Mrs Harding's care with other members of the Primary Health Care Team. Together they will decide whose particular skills could be utilised to help Mrs Harding regain continence (Fig. 9.3).

Test yourself

1   What is the health education role of the District Nurse in relation to incontinence?
2   List the possible causes of incontinence.
3   What aspects of rehabilitation should the District Nurse consider in relation to an incontinent old person?
4   What is the role of the Specialist Nurse Incontinence Adviser?
5   What aids, equipment and services exist in your area that may be useful to an incontinent person?

10 The role of the District Nurse in caring for people affected by HIV/AIDS in the community

This illness, with all its intertwined fears, phobias and stigmas affects the care giver on almost every level of his or her being. This illness challenges the care giver physically, emotionally, spiritually, psychologically, and then only finally professionally. AIDS touches upon the care giver's sense of morality, ethics, humanity and his or her understanding of human rights as well as definitions of compassion and social responsibility.

(Graydon, 1988, p. 67)

How do you feel about AIDS care?

It would not be surprising or unreasonable if you feel anxious or fearful about your first visit to a person with HIV or AIDS. Patients, because of the stage of the epidemic, are most likely to be gay men or intravenous drug users whose lifestyle may be unfamiliar to you or one you disapprove of. Once you meet the patient, however, you will undoubtedly feel better. These patients, more than any others, may have had many bad experiences from both the general public and health care workers and will have fears about your attitude towards their lifestyle, your willingness to touch and care for them and your ability to maintain confidentiality.

Case history

Ben and Darrel, were both 27 years old. They had lived together for five years before Ben became ill and was diagnosed with AIDS. Shortly after Darrel was tested and found to be HIV positive. 'We just held each other and cried, we felt it was the beginning of the end. We were closer than ever before. We were going to fight it together.' Within the year Ben was dying and Darrel cared for him at home. Darrel became a full time care assistant.

'I never thought I had the courage to stomach the things I had to do. I was pleased and proud of myself because I had overcome my own fears. I neglected my own health, but it kept me from going insane with worry and most of all it meant we could be together at home, in private.'

Since they were both so terrified of anyone finding out that they had AIDS they refused District Nursing services. It was not until Darrel became too ill himself to care for Ben that he agreed to accept District Nurses.

'If Ben had been as ill as he was with some other illness – maybe cancer – I am positive we both would not have hesitated to have used the services available, but because it was AIDS the social stigma attached made us, forced us, to remain private and deprived us of the help that could have been available sooner. We were just so afraid of how people would react, even professional people like nurses.'

Stigma and prejudice

A substantial minority of nurses do hold judgmental and homophobic attitudes that affect their practice. Robert Irwin, for example, found that:

The disclosure that a patient is gay, or could be gay, transformed the attitude or behaviour of nurses towards that patient. Homophobia has presented itself in various ways, including – in these days of 'moral panic' – placing high risk stickers on everything from TPR charts to the drip chambers of giving sets for intravenous fluids. Patients have been avoided, ridiculed and exposed to an avalanche of negative and disapproving non-verbal behaviours.

(Irwin, 1992, p. 435)

A study of District Nurses' attitudes (Smith, 1989) found that 97 per cent of the random sample of 50 District Nurses felt that haemophiliacs did not 'deserve to get AIDS'. But they felt differently towards gay men and drug users. A quarter of the sample, for instance, considered that homosexuals 'deserve' to get AIDS and over half suggested that their 'immoral behaviour' had caused the illness. Almost half (47 per cent) said drug users deserved to get AIDS. These sorts of attitudes, even if they are only held by a minority of District Nurses, are enough to threaten our ability to give effective HIV care in the community. As the author of a large national study on community nurses and AIDS care commented that:

Whilst the proportion of staff who were of the opinion that they should have the right to refuse to deal with certain patients were in the minority, they may still give rise to concern. Patients perceptions of nursing staff may depend upon the effects created by negative opinions of such a minority of nursing staff rather than the positive, but often less newsworthy, opinions of the majority. In this event the relationship potential between nurses and patients may suffer.

(Bond, Rhodes *et al.*, 1988, p. 131)

The District Nurse will therefore need to make special efforts to reassure patients and carers that they are accepted. This reassurance is always welcome. Darrel, for instance, having met the District Nurses noted, with evident relief, that:

'They were marvellous, kind, caring and helpful. They couldn't have given a damn what Ben was dying of, he was just another patient who needed care. Why didn't we use them sooner? I wish we had but we were frightened.'

Fear

Many nurses are fearful of 'catching' HIV – even though they know all the facts about how the virus is spread. It is not uncommon for there to be a difference between what we know in our heads and our 'gut' response – people who are scared of spiders know logically that spiders are harmless.

Mode of transmission

- Sex
- Blood
- Mother to child
- Family studies show no social transmission but care is needed

Occupationally acquired HIV is extremely rare! Worldwide over one thousand health care workers have reported high risk incidents, such as HIV contaminated needle stick injury. Less than 1% of these have become HIV positive. The Department of Health Advisory Committee on Dangerous Pathogens (DOH, 1990) noted that there has been **no** seroconversion to date in the 200 incidents reported in the UK since 1986. Nevertheless, the individual District Nurse will have to come to terms with her own assessment of what is an acceptable risk in relation to her duty to care. Do not try to cope on your own – get support! This may mean finding support beyond your friends and family. Some of the nurses most committed to AIDS work are themselves gay and identify closely with gay men who have

HIV related illness. This closeness may be a cause of considerable stress and grief for the nurse. Gay nurses are usually supported in their involvement by their friends and partners. 'Straight' (i.e. heterosexual) nurses, on the other hand, although often equally committed, cannot rely on support from their friends and families. As one District Nurse explained:

> 'My problem was I couldn't talk about it to my husband because he's anti-gay. He told me I mustn't work with AIDS patients because of my responsibility to the kids. Putting myself at risk is one thing, putting my husband and children at risk is another. It's not a simple matter and my relationship is under a lot of strain.'

Ask your District Nurse if there is a local support group for nurses. The stress and burnout in nurses who work with people with AIDS is high but, ironically, can be counterbalanced by becoming involved with AIDS related voluntary associations such as Body Positive or the Terrence Higgins Trust. The good news is that there is a positive correlation between high AIDS work related stress and personal reward, an enhanced sense of self worth, self knowledge and understanding (Guinan, McCallum *et al.*, 1991). There is also a surprising amount of fun.

AIDS care = high stress and high reward

- Nurses face difficult professional, moral and ethical issues
- Fear, that despite all precautions, you may become infected
- The sexual dimension of AIDS makes some nurses uncomfortable
- Family support may be withheld
- AIDS = Accelerated Inner Development Syndrome

Even District Nurses who are committed to caring for people with AIDS and experienced in doing so admit that there are aspects of taking care of AIDS patients that they find 'devastating'. You may feel frustrated at the realisation that nothing you do will ultimately save these relatively young patients from an untimely death. And because of the 'domino effect' of the disease, you may well have to give terminal care to one person and then to his partner and possibly to their friends and/or children. There is a particular need, therefore, for District Nurses caring for people with HIV to 'clarify their purpose'.

The key to successful clinical work with AIDS patients lies in our willingness to look at our own attitudes and fears about death and dying. The feelings of helplessness, loss of control, dependency, uncertainty, and guilt that we experience in working with a person with AIDS require particular attention.

(Smith, 1992, p. 263)

Infection control

Universal precautions should be taken with all patients. Wear a plastic apron and a pair of non-sterile, rubber latex or good quality plastic gloves whenever you anticipate exposure to blood or body fluids, excretions or secretions from any patient. Hand care and intact skin is essential, not only for your protection but equally for your patient's protection. Remember patients, because of their lowered immunity, are at risk from organisms you may carry on your hands. Soiled incontinence sheets can be wrapped in newspaper, double bagged and put in the dustbin. Very hot water and domestic detergent is sufficient to decontaminate household crockery and bedding.

Never resheath needles as this carries a high risk of injury. Always use specially designed sharps bins for waste disposal. If you are collecting blood samples use vacuum syringes. If these are not available, the needle should be removed using a needle holding device before injecting the blood sample from the syringe into the specimen bottle. This avoids the risk of aerosol contamination which can occur if blood is injected back through the needle and the risk of needle stick injury to the person holding the bottle. Districts will have their own procedure following any needle stick accident.

Needle stick injury

- Do not panic!
- Remember occupationally acquired HIV is extremely rare
- Do not suck the injury
- Squeeze out the blood under running water
- Report as soon as possible

Advice and reassurance to carers/family

Family members and other carers have the same fears and concerns expressed by nurses. The District Nurse is in a prime position to identify and alleviate these concerns. Providing information on the mode of transmission of the virus and advice on handling body fluids, household laundry and equipment, will help carers to feel more confident.

Families response to caring for a member with HIV/AIDS

- Fear
- Informed members draw closer
- Social isolation, emotional & physical exhaustion
- Contagious & stigmatising aspects = stress
- AIDS = Actively Involves Distanced Significant others

The constant fear, however irrational, of being contagious and stigmatised creates a degree of stress, social isolation and emotional and physical devastation in family carers that few, if any, other illnesses produce.

Case history: a carer's concern

'People will think they can catch it from us. It's ignorance but, to be fair, we were ignorant until we had to learn more about it, even though it had been on the telly. It wasn't close to home then. It was sensationalised and put on to frighten people and it did frighten a lot of people. So when you're put in the position where you've got to look after someone, you are frightened. It's a death sentence so you've got to be careful. We asked the doctor for a test. He said "You've not been at any risk". But, the thing is, we felt as if we were. And they will think, as we did, that because we've nursed him we must be able to pass it on to them. So we've got to keep it secret.'

The District Nurse is likely to be one of the few people that the carers trust and can share their anxiety with. She is, therefore, in a powerful position to allay irrational fears. She may also encourage the family to join a voluntary agency support group where they can meet and talk to others in the same situation. The role modelling of safe practice by the nurse is not enough to overcome these fears as a number of people assume that nurses who care for people with AIDS must be HIV positive themselves.

Advocacy

The UKCC Code of Professional Conduct notes that the nurse is the patient's advocate and must take steps to prevent any action by another health care worker that could be detrimental to the patient's wellbeing. In relation to HIV testing, for example, the nurse should ensure that the patient has given informed consent and been offered non-directive pre- and post-test counselling.

UKCC 1987, AIDS – testing, treatment and care

Nurses, midwives and health visitors expose themselves to the possibility of civil action for damages or criminal charges of assault if they personally take the blood specimens, and of aiding and abetting such an assault if they knowingly collude with a doctor in obtaining such specimens.

Acting as an advocate for the patient is appropriate in other situations. The patient and/or family may well ask the District Nurse to help them find a sympathetic general practitioner, dentist or funeral director. An important advocacy role for the District Nurse is to support a gay partner's 'next of kin' status vis-à-vis the biological family. This can be particularly problematic if the patient is confused or unconscious and has not made a will or given clear instruction as to whom he wishes to be recognised as next of kin. In fact, many gay men may not realise that the next of kin does not have to be a blood relative. Even if the partner has been nominated as the next of kin by the patient and is therefore recognised as such by the District Nurse, the patient's family may find this difficult to accept.

Case history: after Ben's death

Ben's family, although they had not been in contact with Ben for many years, were shocked and angry that Darrel had organised the funeral and that Ben had left the flat to Darrel in his will. The District Nurse listened to Ben's parents' aggressive words to Darrel. 'We could have accepted you as next of kin if you were a woman, even if you weren't married – but a man! A rat like you – never! We'll take you to court first!' Darrel was in tears but with time and a 'brew' the District Nurse was able to diffuse the situation and reach a more positive conclusion. As Darrel said later:

> 'It was very important for me to be next of kin, because I did feel married to him. I would like to see gay marriages if it would save the wrangle we had at the end. It was a hurtful and humiliating experience. Something a bit more legal has to be sorted out. I was really grateful that the District Nurse was there to explain how I felt – I couldn't have coped alone'.

Encouraging patients to make a will can avoid this situation or at least ameliorate it.

Maintaining confidentiality

Patients, partners and families are more worried about confidentiality – the need to 'keep it secret' – than about almost anything else. This is especially so in relation to being cared for in the community among the people they know. They are aware that other staff in clinics and health centres may see the District Nurse records and may breach confidentiality – if only inadvertently. Avoid writing the words AIDS or HIV on any document or nursing record and do not leave 'cues' to diagnosis such as yellow bags or high risk stickers on view. Remember that information about a person's HIV antibody status is protected under the terms of the NHS (Venereal Diseases) Regulation 1974. Therefore, the patient's express permission to divulge his HIV status must be obtained before this information is given to anyone else. This includes other members of the Primary Health Care Team and the patient's family or partner. If a patient is having unsafe sex with a partner who is not aware of their HIV positive status the 'duty to warn' as opposed to the right of the patient to confidentiality, is a very stressful and ethically difficult dilemma for the nurse.

Case history

> Joe and Mary had been married for ten years. They did not use condoms because she was 'on the pill'. Joe travelled a lot in Africa. Following an attack of oral Candida he was tested positive for HIV. He refused to tell his wife – explaining his illness as exhaustion, and continued to have unprotected sex.

The District Nurse will have to use all her skills to persuade Joe that he should practice safe sex. This will almost certainly mean having to inform Mary of his status. Referral to a counsellor who can help Joe find strategies to do this, with the least damage to the marriage, is advisable.

Keeping 'the secret' continues to be of concern even after the patient's death. The Death Certificate is a public document, available for anyone to look at. Consequently patients, partners and family will not want the words AIDS or HIV to appear on the Death Certificate.

Case history

Fred Brown collected his son's Death Certificate from the G.P. in a sealed envelope. It was not until the Registrar opened it and offered his condolences that the father realised that AIDS was given as the cause of death. He then had to suffer what he considered public humiliation as he used the Certificate to settle outstanding bills and close accounts. A month later he also was dead. His wife said 'He couldn't stand the disgrace of it and died of a broken heart. My life is over. I can't go out and meet anyone because they all know'. The word AIDS on the Death Certificate created a tragedy out of a disaster.

One option open to the G.P. is to enter the cause of death as the opportunistic infection that caused the patients death (for example, disseminated sarcoma, pneumonia or TB) and tick the box on the back of the certificate. This informs the Registrar that more information will be provided on request and ensures that AIDS statistics are accurately recorded, while maintaining the family's confidentiality. There is a debate in progress about whether it is legal to avoid entering the words 'HIV' and 'AIDS' on the Death Certificate. The sheer variety of practices in this matter suggests that it is a 'grey area'. Until people with AIDS and their carers are no longer stigmatised by society it is our duty to act as their advocates and to protect their confidentiality as far as possible. District Nurses should, therefore, discuss the matter of the Death Certificate with the G.P. The patient may even ask the District Nurse to go with him to talk about this to the G.P.

Partnership with patients

> The 'newness' of AIDS and the contemporary expectations of health care among its predominantly young patients have led to the development of 'user friendly', multidisciplinary and truly 'holistic' models of care and an abandonment of paternalism.
>
> (Pinching, 1989, p. 354)

To a large extent this development has been 'consumer led' – the result of articulate patient demand. AIDS patients are experts in the condition and want to be both informed and involved in every aspect of their care. The relationship between the AIDS patient and the District Nurse is one in which the nurse acts as adviser and facilitator and the patients, to a large extent, 'prescribe' the care they want.

Case management

Before you can begin to give care, you must first 'catch your patient'. In the case of AIDS patients, this has not been easy! Few patients choose to be cared for by District Nurses despite the Government's assertion that:

> Caring for AIDS patients in the community is in general the most suitable way of providing treatment and care, not least to assist the patients' wellbeing. It is also important for optimal clinical management and for cost effective utilisation of hospital services.
>
> (Field, 1989, p. ix)

Obstacles to home care

- The patients' views of primary care services
- Primary Health Care Team's knowledge and attitudes to HIV
- Hospital staff's attitude to promoting acceptance of primary care services by their patients

AIDS patients are typically young gay or bisexual men, intravenous drug users and people from high risk areas (such as Africa) and their partners. They lacked knowledge about or confidence in the community services and so they rarely came on the District Nurses' 'books'. In the first five years of the epidemic (1984–1989) the few patients who used the service reported horror stories about yellow bags left on doorsteps and District Nurses in space suits. Not surprisingly patients preferred to use the hospital as their only source of care. As a result many hospital beds were unnecessarily occupied.

Community Liaison Teams or Home Support Teams were set up, usually with a hospital base, to break the cycle described in Fig. 10.1. The Teams use a case management approach, provide information to both patients and hospital staff about community services and train and support statutory and voluntary carers, particularly District Nurses, caring for AIDS patients at home. The Community Liaison or Home Support Team acts as a contact point for the patient and family and as the co-ordinating link between hospital and both statutory and voluntary community services. In effect, they approximate the role of a Liaison Nurse combined with the role of the Macmillan Nurse. The Teams do not do 'hands on care' except in unusual circumstances or to 'fill gaps', for example by providing 24 hour call/cover where this is not available by the local District Nursing service.

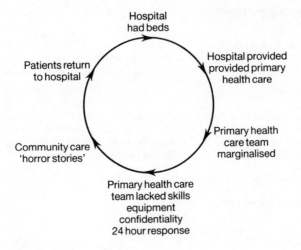

Fig. 10.1   Push/Pull Factions in Community Care of HIV

AIDS home support teams

The aims of these teams are to:

1   Support patients and their carers
2   Increase patient's choice of place of care and death by:
    ● offering symptom control
    ● counselling for both patients and carers
    ● 24 hour on call service
    ● bereavement follow up
    ● education and one to one advice
3   Co-ordinate and support existing services, liaising with hospital and outpatient clinics.

(Butters *et al.*, 1991, p. 59)

Collaborative working, between health authority, local authority, voluntary agencies and the patient, varies between districts from fair to nonexistent. In addition the needs of people with HIV are more diverse than those, say, of the elderly and co-ordinating care is complicated by the erratic and unpredictable nature of the disease and the sudden crises that may arise. Flexible and rapid response home help/carers teams have been set up in some districts to enable dependant patients living alone or with a sick partner to be discharged from hospital. There are still, however, limitations on our ability to care for the demented AIDS patient or those living alone, given that 24 hour care is not, in reality, available in most districts, for more than a couple of days at a time.

*Case management by the Community Liaison/Home Care Team
involves:*

- assessing patient's nursing and social needs
- developing a service plan to meet those needs
- assisting patients in obtaining the services specified in the plan
- monitoring and making necessary adjustments in the service plan as the patient's needs change over time
- offering long-term and flexible support

The heterosexual family

Case history

Joan is a young mother with AIDS. Her husband died a year ago of AIDS. She is trying, with great difficulty, to care for her child with HIV related illness as well as three healthy children. She said 'I have to do it. I want to be in control. I've got to carry my family on. I'm the only person who can really hold my family together, but I couldn't cope without the District Nurse and the Health Visitor'.

The 'domino effect' of AIDS can be particularly devastating in the heterosexual or 'traditional' family.

> 'The whole family can be overcome with despair as it considers the issues and difficulties of living with uncertainty, isolation, death and possible multiple loss. HIV can threaten the very continuance of the family.'
>
> (Kuykendall, 1991)

The District Nurse's priority is to maintain the family as a functioning unit for as long as possible. HIV positive women, who are also carers and mothers often put their responsibilities before their own needs. This is one of the reasons why women present later than men for treatment and may account for the shorter survival time reported for women, as opposed to men.

Over half of the cases reported in Scotland, in contrast to the rest of the UK, are injecting drug users. These families have multiple problems as a result of their drug use, social and economic deprivation and limited family and community support (Reidy, Taggart *et al.*, 1991). In addition, the fear and social stigma of HIV is a major problem as are the attendant difficulties of, for example, having to 'tell the children'. There is, therefore, an understandably high rate of family breakdown and intense stress. Women in such circumstances rely very heavily on the community nurse's support and a study of HIV infected women intravenous users in Edinburgh reported that

'Seventy-five per cent of the women interviewed rated health care professionals as their main source of support' (Bor, 1990, p. 410).

Nursing care

> 'Caring for people with HIV infection or AIDS is not difficult if common sense is applied. No special training is required – simply first class clinical competence, a willingness to learn and to understand, and a desire to care with compassion.'
>
> (Elliot, 1987, p. 106)

Community nurses have already got many of the skills needed to care for people with HIV related illness. You need to bear in mind, however, what makes HIV care different from other conditions.

Features of AIDS which are likely to differ from those of the terminally ill cancer patient

1 Predominantly younger age group.
2 Multi-systems disease which may result in blindness, paralysis, neuropathy, confusion, myopathy, skin disorders and severe diarrhoea.
3 Misery of many co-existing physical problems.
4 Large number of drugs being taken.
5 It is often difficult to identify the terminal phase of the disease – very sick patients may improve and opt for acute treatments.
6 Treatments such as total parental nutrition and intravenous drugs for acute or chronic conditions are given to maintain quality of life in terminal care.
7 Lengthy dying process – patients may be unconscious for a week or more.
8 Most people with AIDS know more about their disease and its treatment than the people caring for them and demand involvement in their care and treatment.
9 Fear, prejudice and lack of compassion are evident in many parts of society.
10 Social isolation of patients and their families.
11 Homelessness or inadequate housing.
12 Need for long-term supervisory care and housing.

(Sims and Moss, 1991)

Patients may be very well for long periods of time and suddenly extremely unwell and dependant. The physical and/or psychological help they perceive themselves as needing and, even more significantly, their acceptance of such help, varies over time. Continuing assessment is therefore necessary and possible if the District Nurse has built up a relationship of trust and visits at regular intervals, even if the patient does not, at that time, require nursing care.

Assessment includes:

Psychological Problems

- Anticipatory grief, sadness, loss, body image concerns
- Anxiety – panic attacks, insomnia
- Anger at injustice/guilt (AIDS = Anger Inappropriately Directed at Self)
- Depression, disturbance of mood, suicide

Physical Problems

- Susceptibility to infection
- Nausea, vomiting, diarrhoea and constipation
- Respiratory distress
- Weakness and fatigue
- Skin problems/breakdown
- Pain
- Confusion, Dementia
- Paralysis
- Blindness

Social Problems

- Stigma
- Loneliness
- Family conflict
- Work and insurance
- Financial problems
- Housing

AIDS has in many ways, become a chronic illness (see Chapter 8) with 'acute' treatment being required intermittently over a number of years. Indeed one of the more obvious distinguishing features of AIDS care is that, although still ultimately fatal there is no clear distinction between the treatment phase and the palliative care phase (Fig 10.2).

AIDS patients are young and see a change from curative to palliative treatment as 'giving up'. Invasive treatment is often continued until very late into the course of the disease. 'Palliation' and 'care' may co-exist – a malignancy may be palliated while an acute complicated infection (e.g. pneumonia) may be treated aggressively to buy time (George, 1990, p. 9).

In the early 1980s the illness often presented as an acute opportunistic infection that led very quickly to death. Improved treatment, however, has led to a significant increase in prognosis and quality of life (George, 1990, p. 8). The mean survival time has doubled since 1987, from ten to twenty months (Peters, Beck *et al.*, 1991). Today people talk about 'living with HIV'. It remains the case, however, that no cure is available and although not conclusively proved, we must assume that people infected with HIV will eventually die from the disease. However, it is notoriously difficult to decide when this 'terminal' stage is reached.

> Patients in an apparently moribund state may recover sufficiently to require rehabilitation not only for themselves physically, but also emotionally for their carers, their families and their friends and partners.
>
> (Sims and Moss, 1991, p. 38)

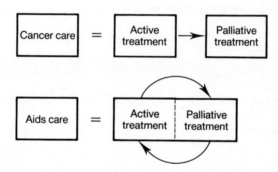

Fig. 10.2   In AIDS care the division between active and palliative treatment is blurred.

Coping strategies

The District Nurse promotes hope in the face of AIDS by 'reminding individuals of the strengths that they possess to cope with difficulties' (Anderson and Wilkie, 1992, p. 153). Creating a positive approach in a situation of uncertainty and loss is aided by the nurse 'just being there' (see Chapters 7 and 8). Providing 24 hour on call contact has been one of the factors enabling patients with AIDS to cope at home.

Case history: Joan's panic attack

'The fact that I knew the District Nurses were there gave me confidence and quite often it meant I did not have to call them.

I will never forget the time I called them, very early on Saturday morning when I was having a panic attack. They came and took over for an hour or two until I was back to normal. After that I didn't have another. I didn't need to, because I knew I had the backup and I knew it worked!'

Symptom control

HIV/AIDS is a state of risk resulting in multi-system diseases and conditions affecting patients' physical, psychological and social wellbeing. Most of these, at every stage of the disease, are amenable to medical treatment and nursing interventions. Health maintenance and good symptom control are, therefore, vital throughout the illness, from the time of diagnosis to terminal care.

Psychological concerns about 'loss' – loss of body image, loss of friends and loss of a future, cause the most demoralising and pernicious symptoms of AIDS. Fear and anxiety accompany every new symptom. It is 'not just one thing, but one thing after another and another and another!' Having AIDS has been described as 'being awake in your own worst nightmare'.

Cytomegalovirus (CMV) retinitis is a common condition in people with HIV which without treatment causes rapidly progressive blindness. Treatment is usually via an established central line and usually six days a week for life. Without District Nurses being willing and able to perform intravenous therapy home care for people with AIDS is a non-starter. As David Edwards has pointed out:

> Where District Nurses are not permitted to administer intravenous medication, patients may be unable to return home, sacrificing quality of life, wasting time and limiting choice.
>
> (Edwards, 1992, p. 18)

The administration of intravenous therapy by District Nurses is important not only for patients unable to administer their own drugs but also as a means of reducing the risk of the central line becoming infected. Research on patients with CMV (Reilly, Nelson *et al.*, 1991) showed that central line sepsis was significantly more frequent in those patients **not** receiving community nurses' supervision and survival was also longer in the supervised group. Although the need for intravenous home therapy is not confined to AIDS patients, it has been the needs and demands of people with AIDS that has acted as the impetus for District Nurses to acquire these skills. In the words of one patient's partner, 'The availability of community nursing over the past twelve months provided the one vital ingredient to enable myself and the family to look after him at home. Together with the District

Nurses we were able to provide a high standard of care to what could be described as acute care'.

The patient's and the doctor's assessment of both the presence of and the distress caused by symptoms do not always agree. A questionnaire study of forty patients and the doctors they had seen in the out-patient clinic found that more symptoms were reported by the patients than by the doctors (Welch, Barlow *et al.*, 1991). The correlation between doctor and patient ratings of the same symptom was generally poor. The symptoms most accurately identified were usually either overt, such as weight loss and skin problems or suggestive of serious disease, such as cough. However, patients were more distressed by such symptoms as anorexia and insomnia. It seemed that when patients had many problems, doctors focused on the most urgent, even though an 'increased awareness of other symptoms may improve the quality of life of these patients'. District Nurses can play a major role in dealing with the symptoms that are of particular concern to patients and affect their quality of life, for example, improving sleeping patterns (see Chapters 7 and 8).

Patients who are depressed or anxious may lack appetite and need encouragement to eat a well balanced, high calorie diet (NACNE and COMA style guidelines are therefore not appropriate (Peck and Johnson, 1990). More commonly, people with HIV are highly committed to maintaining their health and weight at an optimum level as a positive act of self help.

Case history: Paul's story

'I always try to make sure I have a well balanced diet with a good mix of carbohydrate and protein. A substantial part of our income has gone on providing the very best freshest food, prepared and presented with considerable care. This approach has only been partially successful and it must be said that half of the food purchased ends up in the bin. AIDS and medications manage to reduce even the most robust appetite to nil. Many individual meals cost in excess of £10, for the ingredients alone. In normal circumstances this would appear extravagantly wasteful and excessive, but with AIDS eating is a matter of life or death. The success is in the half that is eaten.'

Loss of appetite in a person with HIV may have a number of contributing factors such as alterations in taste (one man who used to love curry now only likes strawberry jam butties), nausea or difficulty in swallowing as a result of oesophagitis. It may be due to a sore mouth caused by aphthous ulceration, gingivitis or oral Kaposi's sarcoma – often exacerbated by the effects of radiotherapy. The most common condition affecting the mouth, however, is *Candida albicans*, a condition any District Nurse would recognise. Unintended weight loss is one of the classic symptoms associated with AIDS patients, indeed 'chronic wasting syndrome', in which the HIV positive patient loses ten or more per cent of their body weight plus either diarrhoea or fever for one month is diagnostic of AIDS. Weight loss may occur as an individual symptom although 'malabsorbtion, diarrhoea, infections and heavy antibiotic treatment, use of inappropriate diets, poor appetite, tiredness, radiotherapy and chemotherapy may compound weight loss (Peck and Johnson, 1990, p. 150). Nutritional supplements are usually recommended by the District Nurse to people with weight loss. Having a liquidizer, a freezer and a microwave makes food preparation easier and can usually be obtained by the District Nurse from AIDS charities.

Nasogastric feeding may be resorted to, in an attempt to slow weight loss when patients cannot meet their nutritional requirements orally. Opportunistic infections such as *Cryptosporidium*, however, result in the production of vast quantities of watery diarrhoea and malabsorbtion. In these patients total parenteral nutrition may be necessary. This is another case in which the ability of the District Nurses to give intravenous infusions at home is an obvious advantage.

Skin problems, are among the most distressing of HIV related conditions, for patients. These include Molluscum contagiosum and fungal infections of the skin and nails such as tinea. Seborrhoeic dermatitis, for example, which is common in the general population is much more severe in HIV, often covering most of the persons face. Itchy folliculitis can 'drive a person crazy' and is very difficult to treat. Likewise dry skin (xeroderma) which is almost universal in AIDS patients is associated with intense itching. The regular use of moisturising creams (e.g. E45 and bath oils) can often give people considerable relief at least from the itching associated with dry skin.

Pain is a frequent symptom experienced by AIDS patients. In some cases it is compounded by the medication. For example, AZT may cause myalgia (muscle pain) and many of the drugs can cause headaches, nausea and gastrointestinal disturbance. Pain can change in severity very quickly.

Case history: Ben's HIV related pain

'Yesterday was a fabulous day but by the evening the pain had started. I took two Temgesic® but nothing seemed enough. It was real pain, it made me feel sick – it was like a knife going in and out. I had to ready myself when I needed to take a breath. It ended up like I was in bits by 4 a.m. When it was at its worst I was in dire agony. The pain killer wasn't strong enough. I couldn't stop crying and it was hurting to cry. When I had that pain I was near to giving up whereas before I was very strong.'

HIV related pains are rarely confined to one area or system of the body or one type of pain and a variety of drugs may be needed to achieve control. Being closely involved with the patient and in a prime position to document the severity, time and duration as well as the location of the pain. District Nurses are well placed to anticipate and differentiate between pains from different causes and to act accordingly. Unfortunately, some common forms of HIV related pain are particularly difficult to control, for example the pain associated with peripheral neuropathy which has been described as 'a blowtorch being run up and down the soles of your feet and legs'.

Alternative therapies

Complementary therapy, is an area in which the District Nurse's interest and knowledge can be crucial in offering some relief from medically minor but irritating conditions which affect the patient's sense of well being. Ben said,

'If nurses used massage it would be brilliant, it would be an enormous benefit to patients. It relaxes you, because you get very tense and worry with one thing and another, it rids you of all that tension. Just half an hour of that physical gentle contact squeezes out all the aches and pains.'

Darrel swears by the essential oil of tea tree (Tisserand, 1988) in an almond oil base to calm his itchy skin and others have followed his suggestion with equal success. In a letter to The British Medical Journal (1989), Barton and his associates published the results of an investigation into the use of alternative and complimentary therapies by 190 patients of the Kobler Centre (formally St Stephen's Hospital), London. The definition of 'alternative' used in the study was 'any treatment not prescribed or supplied by the doctor'. Each patient completed a questionnaire on the use of 15 alternative therapies, including massage, aromatherapy, reflexology, autogenic training, spiritual healing, homeopathy, acupuncture or acupressure, hypnosis, visualisation, vitamin and mineral tablets, herbalism and a number of experimental compounds such as Imuthiol (Hockings, 1988).

Thirty eight per cent of patients reported using at least one alternative therapy following their diagnosis. In total, 20 different types of treatments were cited and 80 per cent of the patients had used 3 or more of them. The authors concluded that:

> The use of alternative treatments reflects the failure of traditional medicine to produce a cure for HIV infection. Furthermore the low rate of reported side effects contrasts sharply with those associated with most drugs taken by patients with HIV infection and may be an important factor in the popularity of alternative medicine.
>
> (Barton *et al.*, 1989, p. 1519)

There are a huge number of alternative therapies offered as treatments for AIDS and the lack of scepticism on the part of some patients may pose problems for the District Nurse. She may 'have to walk a fine line between support for the patient and encouraging him or her to choose foolish and expensive alternative treatments just to foster the patient's sense of autonomy' (White, 1989, p. 12).

Conclusion

> The lack of a biomedical response to AIDS offers nursing the opportunity – probably for the first time since Miss Nightingale's visit to Scutari – to prove what nursing is worth and to demonstrate that although the eventual outcome cannot be changed, the path to the outcome can be made less rigorous and more tolerable through nursing's interventions.
>
> (Pratt, 1988, Foreword p. iv)

Community nurses contribute to both the prevention of the spread of the HIV virus and the treatment and care of people who are HIV positive and their families. Depending on the circumstances certain groups of community nurses will have a more obvious role than others. The person with HIV who is well is most likely to come into contact with the Practice Nurse, for example, for holiday immunisations. Whereas, the person who has HIV related symptoms or is dying of AIDS will need the District Nurse's care. The Community Psychiatric Nurse's skills are obviously useful to people who have depression or HIV related mental illness and/or dementia. The Health Visitors role is primarily with the patient's children, family and the partner/spouse especially if they are also HIV positive. Family Planning Nurses and School Nurses have a vital role in health promotion and HIV prevention and Community Midwives will be increasingly involved with HIV positive mothers and babies as the epidemic spreads. Occupational Health Nurses can support HIV positive people who are working and act as health educators in the work place. The Community Drug Team Nurses may well find that HIV related issues and care will become a central focus of their work.

Role of Community Nurses in HIV/AIDS

- **Information/Support** – with the 'at risk' or 'worried well'
- **Health Promotion** – with the HIV positive patient
- **Prophylactic Treatment** – with the symptomatic patient
- **Symptom Control/Support** – in terminal care
- **Support/Advocacy** – in bereavement

Although, at this stage of the epidemic it is a minority of community nurses who have cared for or knowingly had HIV positive people on their case load, none of us can expect this to be the case for very much longer.

> The number of people who are currently infected with human immunodeficiency virus and who will go on to develop related illnesses indicates that there will come a time in the professional lives of all nurses when they will be faced with the challenge of caring for people with AIDS.
>
> (Pratt, 1988, Foreword p. iv)

Test yourself

1. What are the factors that make AIDS care different from the care of patients with other chronic or life threatening conditions?
2. What should be done in case of accidental exposure to the virus?
3. How is HIV transmitted?
4. Name the AIDS related voluntary agencies in your area and describe their role?
5. What is the health education/promotion role of community nurses in relation to HIV/AIDS prevention and care?

I wish, in the second edition, to acknowledge those people affected by HIV. Above all, I want to thank the people who shared their thoughts and feelings with me and helped me to learn; patients, their partners and families, the staff of the Regional Infectious Diseases Unit at Monsall Hospital, and workers (both statutory and voluntary) in the community.

11 Conclusion

We have only been able to cover some of the aspects of care in the community and in many ways this book raises more questions and issues than it answers. That is the nature of nursing in the community. There are no easy answers and solutions to the problems and needs identified by District Nurses and Health Visitors. The hospital, while important, represents to your patients only a short period in their lives. In essence therefore the community is the real world.

To care in the community is complex. It is to be aware of the influences of many social, economic and political factors which may not be fully apparent in hospital.

In drawing together conclusions there are key issues which we can identify:

1   There is a need for comprehensive liaison between the hospital and the community for many age groups and conditions. In particular we are thinking of the responsibility of nurses working in, for example, Accident and Emergency Departments to be aware of the possibility of child abuse and the need to alert community services. You also need to be aware of the different roles of the community health and social workers and the difficulties of providing services for elderly, chronic, sick or isolated patients on their return home from hospital.

2   Health and social services, while important to the patient, are only a part of the network which supports and cares for people in the community.

3   The family and its relationship to the community is probably the most crucial factor that the District Nurse and Health Visitor have to take into account in their work.

4   There are many variations and patterns of care in the community depending on local needs, and part of your experience will be involved in establishing what services exist and who uses them in your particular area.

5   We have discussed the stress imposed on relatives and friends involved in caring for family members. The work of the District Nurse and Health Visitor is always to help these carers as well as provide nursing for the patient.

6   While the family is the focus for care the Health Visitor has a

responsibility to the wider community in providing health education to groups and in helping communities to be aware of their own health needs.

7   District Nurses and Health Visitors are involved in primary, secondary and tertiary prevention of ill health.

Nursing in the community is clearly not high technology care but essential nursing care and preventive care par excellence. Being intimately involved in peoples' lives over a long period of time, and sharing in the families' sorrows but equally in their joy is what makes nursing in the community a very exciting and satisfying occupation.

References

Anderson, C. and Wilkie P. (1992) *Reflective Helping in HIV and AIDS*. Milton Keynes: Open University Press.

Ashton, J. and Seymour, H. (1985) An Approach to Health Promotion In One Region. *Community Medicine*, 7, 78–86.

Barber, T.H. and Kratz, C. (1980) *Towards Team Care*. Edinburgh: Churchill Livingstone.

Barker, W. (1984) Nutritional Factors: Can They Reduce The Incidence of Mental Handicap? *Health Visitor*, 57(3), 73–7.

Barton, S.E., Hawkins, D.A. *et al.* (1989) Alternative Treatments For HIV Infection (Letter). *British Medical Journal*, 298(6686), 1519–20.

Bauman, E., Brint, A.I., Piper, L. and Wright, A. (1981) *The Holistic Health Lifebook*. Berkley: Berkley Holistic Health Centre Press Inc.

Binney, V., Harkell, G. and Nixon, J. (1981) *Leaving Violent Men: A Study of Refuges and Housing for Battered Women*. London: Women's Aid Federation.

Bond, J., Rhodes, T. *et al.* (1988) *A National Study of HIV Infection/AIDS and Community Nursing Staff in England*. University of Newcastle upon Tyne, Health Care Research Unit.

Bor, R. (1990) The Family and HIV/AIDS. *AIDS Care*, 2(4).

Bowling (1989) Contact With General Practitioners and Differences in Health Status Amongst Elderly People Aged Over 85 Years. *Journal of the Royal College of General Practitioners*, 39, 52–5.

Bowling, A. and Stilwell, B. (1988) *The Nurse In Family Practice*. London: Scutari Press.

Butters E., Higginson I. *et al.* (1991) Community HIV AIDS Teams. *Health Trends*, 23(2), 59–62.

Campbell, B. (1984) *Wigan Pier Revisited*. London: Virago.

Carver, V. (1978) *Child Abuse: A Study Text*. Milton Keynes: Open University Press.

Coloplast Objective Continence (1983) In: Stenhouse, *Objective Continence*. Cambridge: Coloplast Ltd.

Copperman, H. (1983) *Dying At Home*. London: John Wiley & Sons.

Corr, C.A. and Corr, D.M. (1983) *Hospice Care: Principles and Practice*, London: Faber & Faber.

Council for the Education and Training of Health Visitors (1977) *An Investigation Into The Principles of Health Visiting*. London: CETHV.

Cresswell, J. and Pasker, P. (1972) The Frail Who Lead the Frail. *New Society*, May, 407.

Damant (1990) *The Challenges of Primary Care in the 1990s – A Review of Education and Training for Practice Nursing the Substantive Report*. Working Group Report for ENB.

DHSS (1977) *Primary Health Care Teams*, CNO, 77(8).

DHSS (1977) *Prevention and Health Reducing the Risk: Safer Pregnancy and Childbirth*. London: HMSO.

DHSS (1979) *Royal Commission on the National Health Service*. London: HMSO.

DHSS (1980) *A Nutritional Survey of the Elderly at Home*. Report on Health and Social Services, **No. 3 & No. 16**. London: HMSO.

DHSS (1980) *Inequalities in Health: Report of a Research Working Group* (Black Report). London: HMSO.

DHSS (1986) *Neighbourhood Nursing a Focus for Care* (Chair J. Cumberlege). London: HMSO.

DOH (1989) *Report of the Advisory Group on Nurse Prescribing* (Chair J. Crown), London: HMSO.

DOH (1990) *HIV – The Causitive Agent of AIDS and Related Conditions*. Advisory Committee on Dangerous Pathogens. London: HMSO.

DOH (1990) *Working for Patients: Guidance to General Practitioners*. London: HMSO.

DOH (1991) *The Health of the Nation*. London: HMSO.

DOH, Welsh Office, Scottish Office Home and Health Dept and DHSS Northern Ireland (1992) *Immunisation Against Infectious Diseases*. London: HMSO.

Doyle, W., Wynn, A., Wynn, S. and Crawford, M. (1991) Low Birth Weight and Maternal Diet. *Midwife, Health Visitor and Community Nurse*, **27**(2), 44–6.

Draper, P. (1991) *Health Through Public Policy*. London: Green Print.

Duda, D. (1982) *A Guide to Dying at Home*. John Muir Publications.

Dunnell, K. and Dobbs, J. (1982) *Nurses Working in the Community*. OPCS, DHSS.

Edwards, D. (1992) A Team Spirit: A Model of Community Care for People With Late Stage HIV Infection. *Primary Health Care*, **2**(6), 16–18.

Elliot, J. (1987) ABC of AIDS: Nursing Care. *British Medical Journal*, **295** (July), 104–106.

Feldman, D. (1974) Chronic Disabling Illness: A Holistic View. *Journal of Chronic Disease*.

Field, F. (1989) *House of Commons: AIDS Social Services Committee*. London: House of Commons.

Fitzgerald Miller, J. (1983) *Coping With Chronic Illness*. F.A. Davis Company.

Freeman, R. and Heinrich, J. (1981) *Community Health Nursing Practice*. London: Saunders.

Froggatt Report (1988) *Fourth Report of the Independent Scientific Committee on Smoking and Health* (Chaired by Sir P. Froggatt). London: HMSO.

George, R. (1990) Care of Patients with Late Stage HIV Infection and AIDS. *Cancer Care*, **7**(1), 6–10.

Gilmore, M., Bruce, N. and Hunt, M. (1974) *The Work of the Nursing Team in General Practice*, CETHV (reprinted in 1976).

Graydon, D. (1988) AIDS: Observations of a Hospital Chaplain. *Journal of Palliative Care*, **4**(4), 66–69.

Guinan, J. J., McCallum, L. W. *et al.* Stressors and Rewards of Being an AIDS Emotional Support Volunteer. A Scale for Use by Care-givers for People with AIDS. *AIDS Care*, **3**(2), 137–50.

Hall Report (1989/1991) Joint Working Party on Child Health Surveillance.
Hally, M. R. *et al.* (1981) *A Study of Infant Feeding: Factors Influencing Choice of Method Vol 1 and II.* University of Newcastle upon Tyne: Health Care Research Unit.
Health Education Authority (1989). *Birth to Five – A Guide to the First Five Years of Being a Parent.* London: HEA.
Hillier, E. R. (1983) In: Corr, C. A. and Corr, D. M. (Eds.) *Hospice Care .Principles and Practice.* London: Faber & Faber.
Hinton, J. (1979) Comparison of Places and Policies for Terminal Care. *The Lancet,* January 6th.
Hockings, J. (1988) *Walking the Tightrope: Living Positively with AIDS, ARC and HIV.* Loughton: Gale Centre Publications.
HVA and United Kingdom Standing Conference on Health Visitor Education (1992) *The Principles of Health Visiting: a Re-examination.* Health Visitors Association (HVA) & UK Standing Conference on Health Visitor Education.
Irwin, R. (1992) Homophobia in Health Care. *Professional Nurse,* 435–8.
Johnson, M. J. and Werner, C. (1982) We Had No Choice: A Study of Family Guilt Feelings Surrounding Nursing Home Care. *Journal of American Gerontological Nursing,* **8**(11), 61–5.
Kempe, R. S. and Kempe, C. H. (1978) *Child Abuse.* London: Fontana Books.
Knopke, H. J. and Diekelmann, N. (1981) *Approaches to Teaching Primary Health Care.* St Louis: C. V. Mosby.
Kubler Ross, E. (1982) *On Death and Dying.* London: Tavistock.
Kuykendall, J. (1991) Aspect of Psychological Support for Families and Children Affected by HIV. In: Claxton, R. and Harrison, T. (Eds.) *Caring for Children With HIV and AIDS,* pp 146–59. London: Edward Arnold.
Luker, K. (1982) *Evaluating Health Visiting Practice.* London: Royal College of Nursing.
Mandalstam, D. (1980) *Incontinence and Its Management.* Beckenham: Croom Helm Ltd.
McClymont, M., Silvea, T. and Denham, M. (1991) *Health Visiting and Elderly People* (2nd Edn). Edinburgh: Churchill Livingstone.
McIntosh, J. and Richardson, M. (1976) *Work Study of District Nursing Staff.* Scottish Home and Health Department.
NHS Management Executive (1992) *The Health of the Nation – First Steps for the NHS.* London: NHSME.
Oakley, A. (1979) *Becoming A Mother.* Oxford: Robertson.
Office of Population Census and Surveys (1989) *General Household Survey 1986.* London: HMSO.
Office of Population Census and Surveys (1992) *Social Trends* **22.** London: HMSO.
Office of Population Census and Surveys Monitor (1992) *General Household Survey Preliminary Reports for 1991.* **ss92/1.** London: HMSO.
Orr, J. A. (1984) Violence Against Women, *Nursing Times,* **80** (17) (April), 34–6.
Orr, J. A. (1985) Assessing Individual and Family Health. In: Luker, K. and Orr, J.A., *Health Visiting.* Oxford: Blackwell.

Peck, K. and Johnson, S. (1990) The Role of Nutrition in HIV Infection: A Report of the Working Party of the AIDS Interest Group of the BDA. *Journal of Human Nutrition and Dietetics*, **3**, 147–57.

Peters, B. S., Beck, E. J. *et al.* (1991) Changing Disease Patterns in Patients with AIDS in a Referral Centre in the United Kingdom: The Changing Face of AIDS. *British Medical Journal*, **302**, 203–26.

Pinching, A. J. (1989) The Acquired Immunodeficiency Syndrome – What Next. *The Medical Journal of Australia*, **150**, 353–4.

Porter, A. M. D. (1987) The Edinburgh Birthday Card Scheme. In: Taylor R. C. and Buckley E. G. (Eds.), *Preventive Care of the Elderly: A Review of Current Developments*. London: Royal College of General Practitioners.

Pratt, R. J. (1988) *AIDS – A Strategy for Nursing Care*. London: Edward Arnold.

Pritchard, P., Personal Communication.

Reidy, M. Taggart, M. E. *et al.* (1991) Psychosocial Needs Expressed by the Natural Care Givers of HIV Infected Children. *AIDS Care*, **3**(3), 331–43.

Reilly, G., Nelson, M. R. *et al.* (1991) Community Nurse Supervision of Intravenous Therapy in the Community Reduces Line Sepsis and Increases Survival. *British Medical Journal*, (in press).

Robbins, J., (1983) *Caring for the Dying Patient and the Family*. London: Harper & Row.

Robertson, C. (1991) *Health Visiting in Practice* (2nd Edn). Edinburgh: Churchill Livingstone.

Saunders, C. (1983) In: Corr, C. and Corr, D. (Eds.), *Hospice Care: Principles and Practice*. London: Faber & Faber.

Shafer, K. N. *et al.* (1979) *Medical Surgical Nursing*. St Louis: C. V. Mosby.

Short Report (1980) Second Report of the Social Services Committee 1980 (chaired by Robert Short). *Perinatal and Neonatal Mortality* I. London: HMSO.

Sims, R. and Moss, V. (1991) *Terminal Care for People With Aids*. London: Edward Arnold.

Sinfield, A. (1981) *What Unemployment Means*. Oxford: Martin Robertson.

Smallegan, M. (1985) There was Nothing Else To Do: Needs for Care Before Nursing Home Admission. *Journal of American Geriatric Society*, **25**(4), 364–9.

Smith, M. (1989) *Ready, Willing and Able: A Study of Nurses' Attitudes Towards People with AIDS*. DOH, London: HMSO.

Smith, N. (1992) Organising Support for Helpers. In: *Reflective Helping in HIV and AIDS*. Milton Keynes: Open University Press, pp. 261–77.

Smith, P. (1989) Postnatal Concerns of a Mother: An Update. *Midwifery*, **5**, 182–8.

Snelson, W., Mason, L. and Hewitt (1990) Primiparity and Maternal Perceptions, *Health Visitor*, **63**(12), 419–20.

Solberg, S. M. (1985) Indicators of Successful Breastfeeding. In: Houston M. J. (Ed.), *Maternal & Infant Health Care*. Edinburgh: Churchill Livingstone.

Stedeford, A. (1984) *Facing Death*. London: Heinemann.

Talbot, J. (Ed.) (1989) *Infant Feeding: The First Year*. London: Profile Publications Ltd.

Thomas, T *et al*. (1980) *British Medical Journal*, November.

Thompson, M. K. (1980) In: Mandalstam, D., *Incontinence and its Management*. Beckenham: Croom Helm Ltd.

Tisserand, R. (1988) *Aroma Therapy for Everyone*. London: Penguin.

Townsend, P. and Davidson, N. (1982) *Inequalities in Health: The Black Report*. Harmondsworth: Penguin Books.

Twycross, R. G. (1975) *British Medical Journal*, **4**, 212–14.

Twycross, R. G. (1983) Principle and Practice of Pain Relief in Terminal Cancer. In: Corr C. A. and Corr D. M. (Eds.), *Hospice Care: Principles and Practice*. London: Faber & Faber.

UKCC (1990) *Report on Proposals For the Future of Community Education And Practice*. United Kingdom Central Council for Nurses, Midwives and Health Visitors.

UKCC (1992) *The Scope of Professional Practice*. United Kingdom Central Council for Nurses, Midwives and Health Visitors.

Wade and Bowling (1986) Appropriate Use of Drugs by Elderly People. *Journal of Advanced Nursing*, April.

Welch, J. M., Barlow, D. *et al*. (1991) Symptoms of HIV Disease. *Palliative Medicine*, **5**, 46–51.

WHICH? (1983) *What to Do When Someone Dies*. Consumer Association.

White, K. (1989) Alternative Therapies: Counselling Patients About Questionable Treatments. *AIDS Patient Care*, (December), 12–14.

Wilcock, G. K., Gray, J. A. M. and Pritchard, P. H. (1982) *Geriatric Problems in General Practice*. Oxford: Oxford University Press.

Williamson, J. (1981) In: Aire, T. (Ed.), *Health Care of the Elderly*. Beckenham: Croom Helm Ltd.

Wilson, E. (1983) *What Is to Be Done About Violence Against Women*. Harmondsworth: Penguin.

Worden, J. W. (1983) *Grief Counselling and Grief Therapy*. London: Tavistock.

World Health Organisation (1986) *Nursing and The 38 Targets for Health for All*, A Discussion Paper. Copenhagen: WHO Europe Nursing Unit.

Yeates (1972) In: Willington, F. L., *Incontinence in the Elderly*. London: Academic Press.

Zorza, R. V. (1980) *A Way To Die: Living to the End*. London: André Deutsch.

Useful addresses

Age Concern
60 Pitcairn Road
Mitcham
SURREY CR4 3LL

Body Positive
PO Box 493
LONDON W14 0TF 1045

British Diabetic Association
10 Queen Anne Street
LONDON W1M 0BD

Chest, Heart & Stroke
Association
123/127 Whitecross Street
LONDON
EC1Y 8JJ

Child Poverty Action Group
4th Floor
1–5 Bath Street
LONDON
EC1V 9PY

Community Projects Foundation
60 Highbury Grove
LONDON N5 2AG
(Information on Community
Action Projects)

Crusaid
1 Walcott Street
LONDON SW1P 2NG

Disabled Living Foundation
346 Kensington High Street
LONDON W14 8NS

English National Board for
Nursing,
Midwifery and Health Visiting
Victory House
170 Tottenham Court Road
LONDON W1P 0HA

Equal Opportunities
Commission
Overseas House
Quay Street
MANCHESTER M3 4FQ

Foresight: Association for the
Promotion of Preconceptual
Care
The Old Vicarage
Church Lane
Witley
SURREY GU8 5PN

Foundation for the Study of
Sudden Infant Death
15 Belgrave Square
LONDON SW1X 8PS

Gingerbread (The Association
for One Parent Families)
35 Wellington Street
LONDON WC2

Health Visitors Association
50 Southwark Street
LONDON SE1 1UN

Help the Aged
St James Walk
LONDON
EC1R 0BE

(Local Social Services listed
in telephone book under
appropriate Local Authority
name.)

London Lighthouse
111–117 Lancaster Road
LONDON W11 1QT

Marie Curie Cancer Care
28 Belgrave Square
LONDON
SW1X 8QG

National Board for Nursing,
Midwifery
and Health Visiting for Scotland
22 Queen Street
EDINBURGH EH2 1JX

National Board for Nursing,
Midwifery
and Health Visiting for Northern
Ireland
RAC House
79 Chichester Street
BELFAST BT1 4JE

National Childbirth Trust
Alexandra House
Oldham Terrace
Acton
LONDON W3 6NH

National Children's Bureau
8 Wakely Street
LONDON ER1V 7QE

National Council for the
Divorced and Separated
13 High Street
Little Shelford
CAMBRIDGE CB2 5ES

National Council for Voluntary
Organisations
26 Bedford Square
LONDON WC1B 3HV

National Society for Cancer
Relief
30 Dorset Square
LONDON NW1 6QL

National Society for the
Prevention of Cruelty to
Children
Saffron Hill
LONDON
WC1N 8RS

Northern Ireland Council of
Social Services
2 Anadale Avenue
BELFAST BT7 3JR

The Patient's Association
11 Dartmouth Street
LONDON SW1A 9BN

Pregnancy Advisory Service
12–13 Charlotte Street
LONDON W1P 1HD

Queens Nursing Institute
3 Albemarle Way
LONDON C1V 4JB

Relate Marriage Guidance
Herbert Gray College
Little Church Street
RUGBY CV21 3AP
(Local Address in Phone Book)

Royal Association for Disability
and Rehabilitation (RADAR)
25 Mortimer Street
LONDON W1N 8AB

Royal College of Midwifery
15 Mansfield Street
LONDON W1M 0BE

Royal College of Nursing
Henrietta Place
Cavendish Square
LONDON W1M 0AB

Scottish Council for Social
Services
18–19 Claremount Street
EDINBURGH EH7 4QT

S.P.O.D. (Committee on Sexual
Problems of the Disabled)
49 Victoria Street
LONDON SW1

Study Commission on the
Family
3 Park Road
LONDON NW1 6XN
(This is an independent body
which draws together and
analyses information and
research about the family.)

The Terrence Higgins Trust
42–54 Grays Inn Road
LONDON WC1X 8JU

United Kingdom Central
Council for Nursing, Midwifery
and Health Visiting
23 Portland Place
LONDON W1N 3AF

The Volunteer Centre
29 Lower King's Road
Berkhamsted
Herts HP4 2AB
(The national advisory agency
on volunteer and community
involvement.)

Welsh National Board for
Nursing,
Midwifery and Health Visiting
Floor 13
Pearl Assurance House
Greyfriars Road
CARDIFF CF1 3AG

Women's Aid Federation
(England)
PO Box 391
BRISTOL
BS99 7WS

Women's Research and
Resources Centre
27 Clerkenwell Close
LONDON EC1　.

Index